ROUTLEDGE LIBRARY EDITIONS: BRITISH SOCIOLOGICAL ASSOCIATION

Volume 10

HEALTH CARE AND HEALTH KNOWLEDGE

HEALTH CARE AND HEALTH KNOWLEDGE

Edited by
ROBERT DINGWALL,
CHRISTIAN HEATH, MARGARET REID
AND MARGARET STACEY

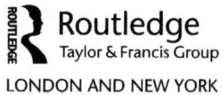

LONDON AND NEW YORK

First published in 1977 by Croom Helm Ltd

This edition first published in 2018
by Routledge
2 Park Square, Milton Park, Abingdon, Oxon OX14 4RN

and by Routledge
711 Third Avenue, New York, NY 10017

Routledge is an imprint of the Taylor & Francis Group, an informa business

© 1977 British Sociological Association

All rights reserved. No part of this book may be reprinted or reproduced or utilised in any form or by any electronic, mechanical, or other means, now known or hereafter invented, including photocopying and recording, or in any information storage or retrieval system, without permission in writing from the publishers.

Trademark notice: Product or corporate names may be trademarks or registered trademarks, and are used only for identification and explanation without intent to infringe.

British Library Cataloguing in Publication Data
A catalogue record for this book is available from the British Library

ISBN: 978-1-138-49942-3 (Set)
ISBN: 978-1-351-01463-2 (Set) (ebk)
ISBN: 978-1-138-48890-8 (Volume 10) (hbk)
ISBN: 978-1-138-48893-9 (Volume 10) (pbk)
ISBN: 978-1-351-03910-9 (Volume 10) (ebk)

Publisher's Note
The publisher has gone to great lengths to ensure the quality of this reprint but points out that some imperfections in the original copies may be apparent.

Disclaimer
The publisher has made every effort to trace copyright holders and would welcome correspondence from those they have been unable to trace.

HEALTH CARE AND HEALTH KNOWLEDGE

Edited by
ROBERT DINGWALL, CHRISTIAN HEATH,
MARGARET REID and MARGARET STACEY

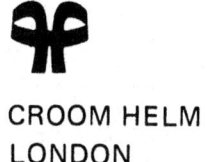

CROOM HELM
LONDON

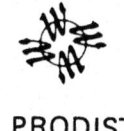

PRODIST
NEW YORK

© British Sociological Association 1977

Croom Helm Ltd,
2-10 St John's Road, London SW11

ISBN 0-85664-482-X

Printed in Great Britain by Biddles Ltd, Guildford, Surrey

CONTENTS

Introduction 9

Images of Pregnancy in Antenatal Literature
Hilary Graham 13

Old Age as a Social Problem *Sally Macintyre* 39

Therapeutic Optimism and Treatment of the Insane
Michael Fears 65

The Reproduction of Medical Knowledge
Paul Atkinson 83

Social Control Rituals in Medicine *Arnold Arluke* 107

Everyday and Medical Knowledge in Categorising Patients
David Hughes 127

Magical Elements in Orthodox Medicine
Tina Posner 141

When Was Your Last Period? *Joel Richman and
W. O. Goldthorp* 160

Policy and Practice in Paramedical Organisations
Malcolm Cross and Sara Arber 185

INTRODUCTION

The 1976 Annual Conference of the British Sociological Association took as its theme 'Sociology, Health and Illness'. In selecting it the intention of the BSA was to reflect the importance of the sociology of medicine in contemporary sociology. The importance of the sub-discipline to the membership of the BSA is reflected in the Medical Sociology Study Group being one of the largest and most active BSA sections. At the same time, the historical neglect of medicine by major sociologists and the past domination of medical sociology by problems and approaches defined in terms set by the medical profession had led to a certain insulation of the sociology of medicine from the mainstream of British sociology. The conference offered an occasion to promote interest in the new directions being developed within the sociology of medicine and to present to the parent discipline some of the theoretical and empirical work available in the field, some of which undoubtedly has implications for the development of mainstream sociology.

Developments in the sociology of medicine have been prompted by both intellectual and social stimuli. On the intellectual side, there was on the one hand the influence of Parsons' seminal insight into the importance of medicine as an element in the maintenance of social order and, on another, the contributions which flowed from interactionist theories of deviance. Medicine has thus come to take its place in the traditional sociological list of control agencies along with education, religion, law and the military. Medicine's claims to value neutrality have been undermined and this has opened the way to enquiries into medicine as a subject of the sociology of knowledge.

Alongside this there have been changes in the social context of medicine. Health care is now a substantial element of most countries' gross national product. It is one of the biggest single industries in any advanced country. Given this, there are inevitably strong pressures for state interest and state intervention to regulate the allocation of national resources to secure the maximum social and economic returns. Relevant information must be collected if the state is to intervene effectively. The expansion of health services has tended to increase with the size of individual institutions and, together with technological change, to modify the traditional division of labour. As health care has become more industrialised, its workers have tended to adopt industrial models of organisation, whether managerial or union. A traditional social order has been disturbed, a phenomenon which has often been a starting-point for sociology.

One must also mention the impact of the feminist critique of medicine. The women's movement has criticised the social processes of health care institutions and the encounters experienced by women in medical settings. Some sociologists have found themselves drawn into an examination of medical encounters through their sympathies with this movement. There has been a wave of research interest in aspects of obstetrics and gynaecology, the implications of which are now being considered for other fields of medicine.

This volume and its companion reflect these new orientations. Here we shall be concentrating on the interface between biological events and social interpretations as we look at the way medical knowledge is developed, transmitted, and brought to bear on particular cases. In this volume interactionist approaches are perhaps dominant, reflecting the balance of work going on in medical sociology at the moment. In the companion volume the work of structuralists is more apparent and more attention is paid to the social and organisational contexts in which interaction takes place. While such a distinction is somewhat artificial, it does lend a certain unity to each of the volumes and defines their mutual relationship. Nowhere, however, among the papers submitted to the conference were problems associated with social class addressed directly or in detail. This remains a gap in both volumes.

As if to illustrate the degree of overlap between the volumes, this collection begins with three papers, by Graham, Macintyre and Fears, which investigate the social and historical contexts against which medical knowledge has developed. Graham and Macintyre tackle this issue at its most general level. In her contribution, Graham reviews the development of a body of popular literature dealing with pregnancy in the light of changing conceptions of the nature of women and of their place in society. She contrasts the growing romanticism of the popular literature with the crudity and harshness of more technical material, especially on the processes of birth and ante-natal care. Despite all the images which are presented to women there is nothing romantic about medicalised parturition. Macintyre uses government reports to examine changing conceptions of the elderly. She traces the interplay of humanitarian concern for old people's welfare and organisational convenience, usually financial, as expressed in the shifts of state policy from the days of the workhouse to the present emphasis on community care. Fears, in contrast, takes a specific historical period and a single institution in order to study the emergence of medical knowledge. In analysing the origins of Tuke's therapy for the insane at the Retreat, he allows us to see the development and implementation of new ideas at an institutional level as a counterpoint to the more generalised discussions of the earlier papers.

Fears is concerned with the emergence of medical knowledge, but Atkinson and Arluke are both concerned with its perpetuation as it is transmitted to novices. They both demonstrate the importance of the clinical context in such a process. Atkinson shows how the general body of knowledge which medical students are expected to acquire is specifically realised through the teaching activities of the clinician. Arluke's paper looks at the response to the disorder created for these general schemes by the intervention of death. The efficacy of the physician's working knowledge is restored by the collective agreement that he had done everything he could.

Hughes and Posner both explore the use of medical knowledge in order to assess its precise nature and status. In her paper on the management of diabetes, Posner shows the continuities between 'magical' and 'scientific' thinking. This traditional distinction has come under increasing attack from philosophy, anthropology and sociology in recent years as the claims of science to objective knowledge have been investigated. Scientific and medical knowledge may be seen as just another set of ideas validated by social consensus. Once this is accepted, then, as Posner shows, they become susceptible to the same kind of analysis and display the same features as magic. Hughes' work on a casualty department provides some suggestions for alternative ways of thinking about knowledge as he probes the interdependence of commonsense and scientific thinking in the activities of departmental staff. He stresses how ordinary is the character of much of the reasoning behind diagnosis and treatment. While neither of these papers explores in detail the consequences of their critique of the claims of medical knowledge, they do clearly show how untenable is the notion of a sharp distinction between that and other types of knowledge.

The final selections in this volume examine the work of patients in medical encounters. Richman and Goldthorp examine the management of time in gynaecological consultations. Time is a neglected dimension of social life yet, as a finite resource in the life of any individual, it is surrounded by a network of rights and obligations which organise and structure its passage. Richman and Goldthorp describe the distribution of temporal rights in one type of medical encounter and the ways in which this provides for the actions of both consultant and patient. The running of the clinic is seen to depend on assigning a nil value to patients' time. In the final paper on family planning in Trinidad, Cross and Arber show how the efficacy of this programme is limited by the constraints deriving from the priority given to medical definitions of the situation over those of clients. There are similar assumptions of a nil value on clients' time, of a lack of preference by clients for any particular method and an assumption that all clients who cease to attend are irrational. Yet, as Cross and Arber demonstrate, there are competing demands on clients' time; clients do have definite and reasonable preferences of method, based on their experience of side effects and some clients will inevitably cease to attend because they plan to get pregnant or they reach the menopause. Blaming the client without questioning the structure of the delivery service achieves little.

The particular issues raised in each paper will be taken up in our introductions to each. The central theme of the volume remains, however, that biological events are not immutable facts. They take on their significance for social life only through organised acts of perception, interpretation and formulation. In a variety of ways, this position underlies all of these papers. It proclaims the emancipation of medical sociology from a medical model of biological events and the transformation of medical sociology into a sociology of health and illness which can reflect upon that medical model as just one among a number of ways of describing health, illness and treatment. In adopting this stance, the sociology of health and illness can find a secure ground from which to assess the social implications of health service policies and practices.

RD, CH, MR, MS.

Hilary Graham's paper analyses the changing theories about the nature of pregnancy which have been presented to women through popular advice literature. It contains both a historical and a contemporary dimension. Vernacular accounts of childbearing first became available only during the sixteenth century, although one may dispute whether this was due to medical prudery, as Graham suggests, or due to a general dearth of material in English prior to the introduction of printing and the secularisation of book production. Whatever the reason, these accounts were intended almost exclusively for midwives and, later, obstetricians; only in the early nineteenth century did a genuine popular literature emerge with the publication of a number of books interpreting medical theories for the general population of pregnant women.

Graham describes and analyses the images of pregnancy embodied in this literature and sketches in its social background. Reproduction became a major social issue in the latter part of the nineteenth century under the sponsorship of eugenicists and Social Darwinists who were disturbed by perceived threats to the quality of the British race. They saw degeneracy everywhere, in the crises of morale provoked by the emergence of a commercial competitor in Germany, by the rising influence of socialist movements among the working class, by severe epidemics and, towards the end of the century, by the military debacle of the Boer War. This degeneracy was attributed to the declining birth-rate of the middle and upper classes and to the high birth-rate of the working classes. The race was being perpetuated by its least fit members. These worries stimulated a number of interventionist movements directed at both ante- and post-natal care. They had the twin aims of controlling the class imbalance in birth-rates and of improving the quality of surviving children by measures designed to reduce infant mortality and morbidity. This antenatal literature directed at literate women, which still meant largely the middle and upper classes, was intended to persuade them of their patriotic duty to bear children and to ensure their health.

These themes changed little until comparatively recently. Since the Second World War, a new romanticism has emerged, largely under the influence of the pre-war writings of Grantly Dick Read. Although these still contain eugenicist elements, they mark a reversion to a spiritual emphasis in ante-natal care. Pregnancy becomes an almost mystical experience. In the latter part of her paper Graham contrasts this romanticism and its potency in contemporary popular literature with the gritty realism of more technical material. The latter may correspond more closely to the practical experience of pregnancy and childbirth, but in it they are not portrayed with the potent symbolism of popular literature. The consequence, Graham implies, is that women may be poorly prepared for the harsh realities of high-technology childbirth. The idealism of their expectations may magnify, if not create, the shock and distress which many seem to experience. Such a suggestion can, however, only be answered in the context of further research on the ways in which women actually make sense of the social and physical experiences of pregnancy and childbirth.

R.D

IMAGES OF PREGNANCY IN ANTENATAL LITERATURE

Hilary Graham

The observation is often made that child-rearing has become a major cultural preoccupation in Western society. This particular predilection has been explored in some depth by social scientists and historians, with several studies charting its historical evolution and the present-day patterns of attitudes and practices.[1] Such studies have drawn attention to a distinctive feature of the contemporary approach to parenthood, namely the reliance upon specialist knowledge gleaned from outside the traditional family and community networks. This professional guidance is provided through contact with the socially appointed experts, the doctor, the health visitor, the social worker, and, more particularly, through an increasing proliferation of sophisticated books, magazines and leaflets, complemented by educational programmes on television and radio.

This popular literature on child care has recently become a subject of analysis in its own right, studied not so much for what it reveals about scientific theories nor for what it tells us about the empirical patterns of child-rearing, but from the assumption that it contains a distillation of cultural understandings about the nature and management of children.[2] This kind of analysis could also be made of literature relating not only to child care, but also to its biological antecedents of pregnancy and childbirth. Historically, advice material on the process of reproduction reveals a pattern of development related to the emergence of child care pedagogies, with the style of antenatal guides adapting in parallel to but slightly later than, literature which focused on the years after birth. The form and content of these publications can be similarly seen as expressive of the cultural climate relating, in this case, not so much to children as to women and their reproductive role. However, despite the recent proliferation of books and magazines, films and commercials on child-bearing, this material has remained, sociologically, an untapped resource.

The paper seeks to remedy this omission of popular printed material on pregnancy. It does not consider literature on childbirth, which is now, in many respects, an autonomous sub-speciality within the mass media. However, many of the observations made about the portrayal of pregnancy can, by extension, be applied to the media's treatment of childbirth which appears to bring out, in stronger relief, the same themes as those evident in antenatal literature. These themes seem to revolve around the nature of child-bearing and focus particularly on the question of whether or not pregnancy and childbirth are, and can be treated as, natural processes. Although the major authorities agree that pregnancy is a 'natural function' and 'a perfectly normal event', where mothers enjoy 'the best of health' and feel 'an immense sense of achievement and satisfaction', they invariably qualify this position in various ways.[3] Pregnancy may be healthy but is 'often bedevilled by a whole variety of minor ailments . . . morning sickness, heartburn, piles and constipation, faintness and dizziness, varicose veins'.[4] Similarly, pregnancy may be a 'normal physiological process' but nonetheless expectant mothers are advised, in another popular guide, that 'There is an extremely close relationship between the physical and the psychological and some women will undergo a profound change in their emotional state as well as their psychological balance.'[5] Again, although a natural condition, readers are instructed to 'visit your doctor or midwife regularly . . . listen carefully to the advice your doctor and midwife give you . . . and (follow) doctor's orders'[6]

Such information and advice, evident in most antenatal literature, suggests that their initial characterisation of pregnancy as natural, normal and healthy is ambiguous in several respects. There is ambiguity apparent in the depiction of pregnancy as firstly both healthy *and* a time of sickness; secondly as physiologically normal *and* emotionally stressful; and thirdly as both natural *and* medically problematic.

It is interesting that an ambiguity concerning the status of pregnancy is not peculiar to contemporary antenatal guides. Rather a confusion about its relation to health and pathology, to physiology and psychology, and to nature and medicine, represents a continuation of an historical dialogue which I was able to trace back to the earliest advice literature for expectant mothers. appearing in the first decades of the nineteenth century. Because of the relevance of an historical perspective, I attempt to map out the ideas about expectant motherhood in two ways:

(1) by looking at the historical development of a popular literature on pregnancy in terms of these types of uncertainty about its nature and status;

(2) by considering the way these themes are apparent in the images of expectant motherhood contained in contemporary material.

The Historical Development of Antenatal Literature

Women, whether in the role of expectant mother, or in the role of midwife, have historically had limited access to the available scientific knowledge on the child-bearing process. The prohibition against the dissemination of information to a lay audience, and midwives as well as mothers were placed in this category, was not solely related to the sense of prudery and propriety which surrounded matters of a sexual nature. The taboo against the discussion of either the anatomy or the management of reproduction also derived from the general attitude of Western medicine towards medical care which involved physical contact with the patient's body.[7] While in the Middle East, information on pregnancy and childbirth was apparently available from 2200 B.C., in Britain medical advice for the midwife was effectively withheld until the sixteenth century by the publication of textbooks in Latin. It was not until 1540 that a midwifery annual, 'the Byrth of Mankinde', was published in English, a development which was not altogether welcomed. In fact the prologue to the work contained the following apology: 'Many thinke it not meete ne fitting that such matters be intreated of so plainly in our mother and vulgar language to the dishonour of womanhood and the derision of their secrets.'[8]

The notion that it was irreverent, and subversive, to publish information about the intimacies of the female body was not quashed with the publication of 'the Byrth of Mankinde'. For example, a translation of a French midwifery textbook published over a century later, in 1673, omitted the anatomical drawings included in the French original on the grounds that 'there being already severall in English; and also here and there a passage that might offend a chaste English eye'.[9]

This opinion was taken further in another seventeenth-century work, which excluded any illustrations and descriptions of what it called 'the parts destined to generation' because the writer felt such information was not 'absolutely necessary' in a midwifery textbook. Further, the author suggested that 'it might seem excreable to the more chast and shamefaced through bawdiness and impurity of words'.[10]

In the course of the late eighteenth and early nineteenth centuries, there appears to have been a relaxation of this puritanical attitude, for descriptions of gestation and birth became less euphemistic and the pathological potentialities of child-bearing were spelt out in more detail.[11] In many ways, the midwifery manuals of this period were a repository of what today are denigrated as old wives' tales, although their emphasis upon morbidity and mortality was consistent with the reality of child-bearing at the time. One popular text, first published in 1792, offered the following advice to midwives: 'A woman, after conception, during the time of her being with child, ought to be looked upon as being indisposed or sick, though in good health; for child-bearing is a kind of nine months sickness ... A woman with child is often in danger of miscarrying and losing her life ...'[12] Other nineteenth-century writers expressed similar sentiments: 'Pregnancy is a physiological state but one bordering so closely upon the pathological that it is sometimes difficult to point out the boundary between them.'[13]

Pathology resided not only in pregnancy but in any condition whose cause could be linked to the woman's possession of a uterus, which, according to a text published in 1828, was 'the great centre of influence in the female system'.[14] A law of sympathy between the uterus and the rest of the body was postulated as the cause of the physiological and psychological symptoms associated with pregnancy, with such disorder as fainting, hysteria and depression explained as an emotional manifestation of the excited condition of the womb. These disorders were seen to be exacerbated by the state of plethora which apparently existed during pregnancy as a result of the build-up of menstrual blood in the system, and could only be averted by active medical intervention − through the practice of bleeding, frequently by the application of leeches, and through the administration of purgatives and sedatives.[15]

Because of the intimate interplay between mind and body, during pregnancy, the expectant mother and her child not only faced physical dangers from 'violent motions ... lifting her arms too high or reposing herself on hard and uneasy seats',[16] but also was vulnerable to sights, sounds and emotions which could threaten the course and outcome of pregnancy. As one nineteenth-century author noted: 'Let no one present any strange or unwholesome things to her, not so much as name it, lest she should desire it and not be able to get it and so either cause her to miscarry or the child to have some deformity on that account.'[17]

The idea that pregnancy was a period of physical and psychological vulnerability was not, it seems, limited to medical texts, but was part of the social ambiance regarding child-bearing.[18] It was into this context that the first advice books for expectant mothers were introduced at the beginning of the nineteenth century — two hundred and fifty years after printed material became available to midwives.[19] Although the new books, Chavasse's *Advice to a wife on the management of her own health*, published in 1832; Thomas Bull's *Hints to Mothers* (1837); George Black's *Young Wife's Advice Book* (1880), reflected medical theories about the aetiology of the disorders associated with pregnancy, they interpreted these findings in a subtly different way. The argued that the side-effects which made pregnancy pathological were invariably caused by the expectant mother excessively stimulating, through drinking and overeating, through dancing and late nights, the organs in sympathetic influence with the uterus. Pregnancy, the Victorian writers maintained was a 'natural process and NOT a disease'.[20] Ill health, including miscarriage and stillbirth, resulted from self-induced invalidism and the overindulgence of bodily needs. The achievement of health thus depended, not upon medical intervention as advocated in the nineteenth-century obstetric texts, but rather upon a regular and restrained approach to diet, defecation, fresh air and sex which would bring the woman's daily life into harmony with nature. This superiority of nature over medicine in controlling the child-bearing process was a constant theme in the health guides. For example, Dr Chavasse in his 1832 manual declares: 'Nature is perfectly competent to bring without the assistance of man, a child into the world . . . Assist Nature! Can anything be more absurd? As though God in his wisdom . . . required the assistance of man.'[21] Although the health writers condemned medical interference and the indulgent attitude to the expectant mother's whims and fancies, they nonetheless recognised that pregnant women required special types of protection. In particular, they stressed the role of emotions in determining the course and outcome of pregnancy. In discussing this psychological dimension, Dr Black notes:

> . . . constant worry and anxiety are hurtful and so are all those sounds and sights which strongly impress the mind. They are bad for the pregnant woman and alike bad for the child in her womb . . . and anything that is known to operate in the way of causing mental shock, mental depression or excitement should be scrupulously avoided.[22]

Although the Victorian advice writers accepted the traditional orientation to the role of psychology in pregnancy, their philosophy as a whole, with its emphasis upon self-determination and health rather than passivity and invalidism offered the expectant mother an alternative to the older pathological model of pregnancy espoused in the midwifery texts. However, this emphasis came not as one might expect from a humanitarian concern for the expectant mother's health and happiness, but rather from an eugenic interest in the quality of her child. It is this eugenic orientation that helps explain the introduction of sex education manuals into a female market which had traditionally been restricted to books on moral enlightenment and the virtues of femininity.[23] In this respect the inspiration, and the legitimation, for the early antenatal literature was similar to that which underpinned the nineteenth-century manuals on child care and derived from an increasing recognition of the role of parental behaviour in securing the mental and physical well-being of the future generation. In the case of pregnancy, it was the recognition of the pre-natal determinants of infant morbidity and mortality that was particularly crucial.[24] Thus one popular nineteenth-century writer justifies his treatise on pregnancy as follows:

> By making a wife strong, she will not only, in the majority of cases be made fruitful, but capable of bringing *healthy* children into the world. This latter inducement is of great importance for . . . it is the children of England that are to be her future men and women — her glory and her greatness! How desirable it is then that her children should be strong and healthy![25]

The eugenic orientation to pregnancy, where a concern with the child legitimised the extension of the principles of child care to cover the pre-natal period, becomes more evident in the publications which gradually replaced the Victorian health books in the second decades of this century. Among the new guides were Frederik Truby King's *Expectant Mother and Baby's First Month* (1922), a companion volume to his *Feeding and Care of Baby*, and Mabel Liddiards's *Mothercraft Manual* (1924), which provide exemplars of the philosophy of pregnancy advocated in early twentieth-century literature. Like their Victorian predecessors, both writers maintained that pregnancy is 'a natural and normal event and not a disease'. 'It is only the effect of civilisation that has brought about the thought that it is an illness.'[26] Within the same basic perspective, shifts of emphasis are nonetheless apparent in those twentieth-century manuals. The guides display a concern not only with the proclivities of an indolent elite but with the poor, whose health was seen as essential to securing the survival of the nation.[27] Their texts reveal a widening medical jurisdiction over pregnancy, a jurisdiction which was receiving, at the time, both political and legal encouragement.[28] Reflecting these trends, Truby King, for example, in addition to reiterating the Victorian theme of the patriotic responsibilities of the mother to her unborn child declares (in a section entitled 'the destiny of the race in the hands of its mothers') that eugenics is a political as well as an individual concern. 'Today our historians and politicians think in terms of regiments and dreadnoughts: the time will come when they must think in terms of babies and motherhood. We must think in such terms, too, if we wish Great Britain to be much longer great.'[29]

There are other amendments to the Victorian model. The writers adopt a more authoritarian style, laying down 'laws of health', 'commandments' and 'rules' rather than offering 'hints' and 'advice'. The difference in vocabulary reflects a more fundamental change in approach: from an emphasis upon self-control to one upon medical control. The puritanical philosophy is no longer couched in the quasi-religious morality of the Victorian advice writers but in a scientific morality where it is the doctor rather than God and nature who is omnipotent. Thus one handbook notes (the italics in original):

> It is no exaggeration to say that, armed with the new knowledge available, it is now possible for practically every mother to go through her confinements in *perfect health.*
>
> Obstetrical science has reached the point where baby can be kept down to the exact weight nature intended him to be, where mother gains no more and no less than she should, where the actual birth is safe and painless ... The obstetrician, with the sum total of decades of research at his finger tips can achieve these pleasant results – not part of the time, but barring unusual conditions, *in every case.* There's only one stipulation, but it's a vitally important one – *obey your doctor* and see him often.[30]

Obeying your doctor involved paying meticulous attention to personal hygiene – in particular to diet and mastication and to the excretory organs which had to be 'kept in good working order'. This obsessive concern with matter introduced and eliminated from the body derived from the hygienist's stress upon purity of the blood. It was according to Liddiard: '... upon the purity and health-giving qualities of the blood that the future health of the child will be to a large extent determined'.[31] Constipation, bad teeth, poor mastication, unhealthy skin could all result in the transmission of impurity to the unborn child, as could the consumption of alcohol, which, Truby King maintained 'flows as a poison in her blood. The tender growing cells of the baby, directly nourished by this poisoned stream ... do not grow or develop properly; they become stunted and degenerate.'[32]

In this physiological orientation, the hygienists had little time for a discussion of the moods of pregnancy which absorbed the Victorian writers. Truby King briefly discusses the notion that maternal emotions can influence foetal development in a chapter entitled 'Popular Errors', dismissing the theory as a 'silly worry'. In the same section, he rejects the view that pregnancy is a time of mood changes and invalidism with the comment: 'Nothing of the kind. The pregnant woman should be radiantly healthy, happy and uplifted.'[33] In a similar vein he notes that 'miscarriage is an evidence of weakness and lack of tone. The tendency to drift into a state of passive invalidism must of all things be avoided, as nothing tends more surely to miscarriage than a state of feeble flabbiness.'[34]

This austere and authoritarian philosophy of pregnancy, with its emphasis on physiology, health and medical control, did not, however, go unchallenged. Within a decade of the publication of Truby King's 'Expectant Mother and Baby's First Month', an English obstetrician, Grantly Dick Read, brought out his book on natural childbirth.[35] While the writings of Truby King had clear links with the philosophy of the Victorian health enthusiasts, Dick Read introduced a new, non-eugenic dimension into the public discussion of pregnancy. Instead of being simply an adjunct to motherhood, Dick Read argued that pregnancy was a condition with its own qualitative distinctiveness, where maternal welfare as well as foetal health must be safeguarded.

This divergence between the two pedagogies can be conceived as a disagreement over what was to be meant by, and included in, the term 'natural'. Both Truby King and Dick Read, like their Victorian forebears, identified pregnancy as a 'natural process' and not a disease; both glorified breast feeding as the 'natural food'. Truby King spoke of the body's 'natural functions' and Dick Read named his first book 'natural childbirth'. But while to the former, nature referred to physiology, to the later it was a psychological state. As if in dialogue with Truby King, Dick Read states: 'I am far more concerned that you should have no doubts or fears on your mind than I am about your health. Your body is much less likely to mar your happiness just now than your mind is.'[36] Thus while Truby King saw natural child-bearing as something achieved by obedience to a set of inviolable scientific laws, Dick Read emphasised that personal understanding coupled with medical non-intervention were the prerequisites of a natural pregnancy and childbirth.

In his recognition of a psychological dimension to pregnancy Dick Read revived some of the nineteenth-century's theories. For example, he saw the side-effects of pregnancy — morning sickness, lassitude, food cravings — as sympathetic physiological reaction to the woman's nervous system. He also reinstituted some of the mysticism which traditionally surrounded the pregnant woman, acknowledging and accepting her emotional lability, her 'acuteness of mind and thought', the perversities of her appetite and the strange mental powers she had over her unborn child.[37] In this context, Dick Read discusses the role of the husband, who, for the first time in antenatal literature, is cast as an important actor in the drama of pregnancy. According to Dick Read, it is the husband, rather than the doctor, who holds the key to a happy and healthy pregnancy; for the expectant mother 'can be happy only if her husband shares her hopes and her anxieties, her laughter and her waves of fear. He alone can be the safety valve of her unpredictable emotions and accept unmoved the explosions of her love, hate, fear, jealousy and anger.'[38]

Although chronologically belonging to the mid-twentieth century, Dick Read's revolutionary philosophy, with its emotional orientation and its antipathy to medicalised child-bearing, was largely rejected by the medical establishment of the time.[39] Instead, the organisation of obstetrics and the style of popular advice books reflected the kind of asepticism and authoritarianism advocated by Truby King. However, as the century progressed, the hygienist influence upon the scope and content of antenatal literature diminished, and from about the late '50s, the themes of Dick Read's early writings began to be revived in the popular press. In the space of six or seven years, between about 1958 and 1964, over a dozen psychoprophylactic guides to pregnancy and childbirth were published in England, several of which are still best sellers today.[40] At the same time, two specialist monthly magazines — *Mother* and *Mother and Baby* — began to offer regular advice on both the emotional aspects of pregnancy and on natural childbirth, and the British Medical Association launched a series of Family Doctor Publications on child-bearing, one of which — *You and Your Baby* —

is today, in an updated edition, the most widely read of the antenatal guides.[41] In these booklets, the principles of psychoprophylaxis were — and are — portrayed not as a radical alternative, but rather as a practical complement to medical practices during pregnancy and childbirth. Unlike the feminist material on child-bearing, the popular guides have extracted from Dick Read's writing the breathing and relaxation techniques and employed them as ameliorative strategies to enhance the mother's experiences of a hospital-based and pharmacological confinement. Although ostensibly acknowledging the principles of natural childbirth, the concern with psychology and individual control is subsumed by and lost within a system of maternity care which, instead, stresses physiology and medical control.[42] Thus, unlike previous advice writers, whose philosophies were internally consistent in their emphasis on psychology and self-management or on physiology and active medical involvement, today's popular authors simultaneously espouse two models of child-bearing. They are committed on the one hand to the ideological veneer of natural childbirth, with its orientation to maternal emotions, individual understanding and medical non-intervention, and on the other to a model of pregnancy which, although consistent with the reality of antenatal care, systematically thwarts psychoprophylactic goals.[43]

Developments in the use of illustrative techniques in antenatal guides coincided with the development of this new, dualistic approach to child-bearing, where a psychodynamic dimension is grafted on to a physiological model of pregnancy. Illustrations of pregnancy had traditionally been kept to a minimum in popular material, and where drawings were included their purpose was invariably instructive — showing the workings of the abdominal binder, demonstrating various styles of antenatal exercises — and the models were demonstrably not pregnant. However, from the early sixties, two developments — the introduction of photographs and the use of pregnant models — have transformed the look of ante-natal literature. Since then, photographs of expectant mothers and women in childbirth have been featured in the cinema [44] and in books [45] — and gradually even in that more conservative barometer of social change, women's magazines.[46]

The introduction of photographs has not just brought a realism and colourfulness to antenatal literature. It has, in addition, introduced another dimension to being pregnant. While drawings continue to emphasise the physiological and medical aspects of pregnancy, photographs seem to represent, in a romanticised way, the kind of psychologistic perspective advocated by Dick Read. In other words, it seems that the historical ambiguities concerning physiology and psychology, and nature and medicine are played out in the illustrations that accompany the popular guides through the use of different visual forms. The third area of ambiguity — concerning health and sickness — is less explicitly developed, perhaps because although the positive and health-giving aspects of pregnancy lend themselves better to visual representation, scenes of morning sickness, heartburn and depression are practically — and aesthetically — less amenable to illustration.

Rather than examining the way these three sources of uncertainty are tackled in the written accounts of pregnancy given by contemporary authorities, it is interesting to consider the way they are managed at a visual level, through drawings and photographs. This analysis has been considerably facilitated by Trevor Millum's recent book, on images of women in advertising,[47] and it is his type of approach which underpins the following section.

Illustrations of Pregnancy in Modern Antenatal Literature

Modern antenatal guides frequently contain pictures of pregnant women, both in their texts and in the accompanying advertisements. Two of these pictures, fairly typical of the style of antenatal illustrations, are reproduced in Figures 1 and 2. Fig. 1 is taken from a DHSS leaflet, *You and Your New Baby*; Fig. 2 is included in the most popular of the antenatal publications, the Family Doctor book, *You and Your Baby*, and, like the DHSS guide, is distributed free through antenatal clinics and doctors' surgeries.[48] Neither picture has an advertising function, but appear in the main text of the respective guides. Despite their similar non-commercial role, there are certain differences in the design and composition of the two illustrations. Describing them in terms of iconographic criteria, we can simply say that one is a drawing and the other is a photograph. If we categorise them according to their form, their overall design, we find one illustration, the drawing, has two-tone colouring and is crowded and somewhat old-fashioned in appearance while the other, by contrast, is colourful, uncluttered and modern looking. Distinguishing between the illustrations according to content elaborates these differences. In Fig. 1, we find the model is engaged in an activity — she is seen visiting her doctor. Other drawings in antenatal guides reveal the models in similarly activity-orientated pursuits — doing exercises, seeing the midwife, or watching their diet.[49] In Fig. 2, the pregnant woman is doing nothing, a pose found

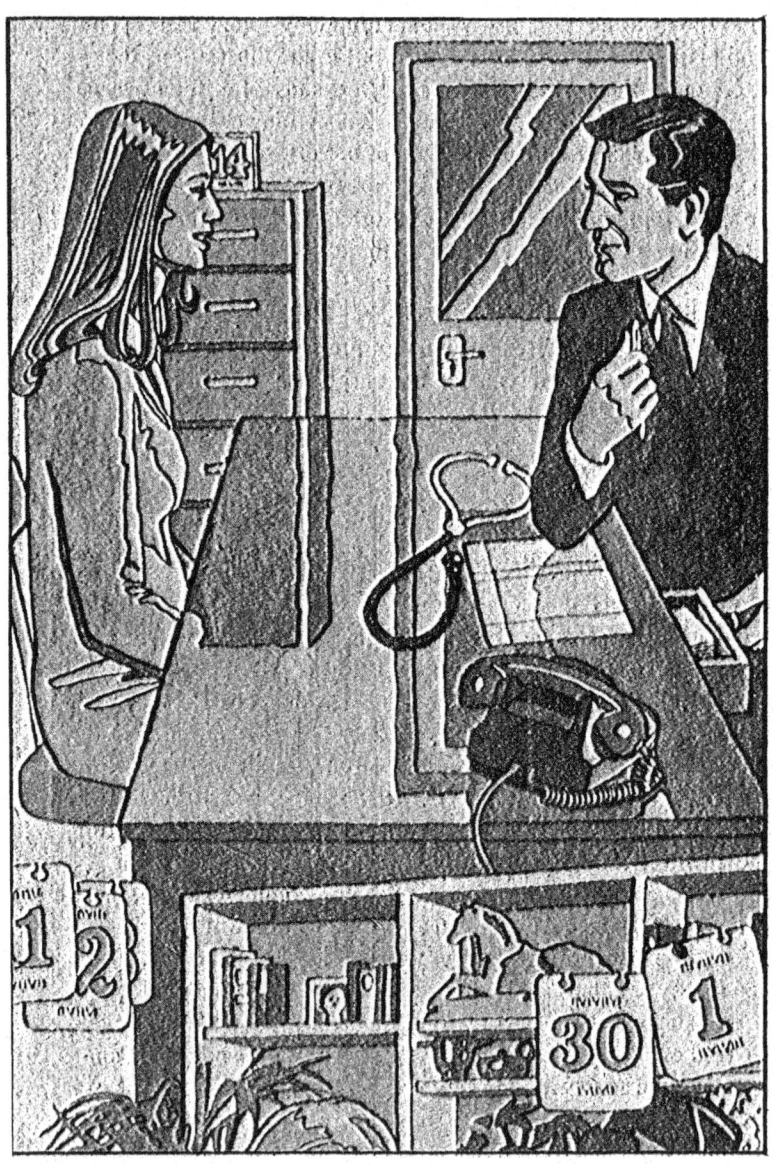

Fig. 1

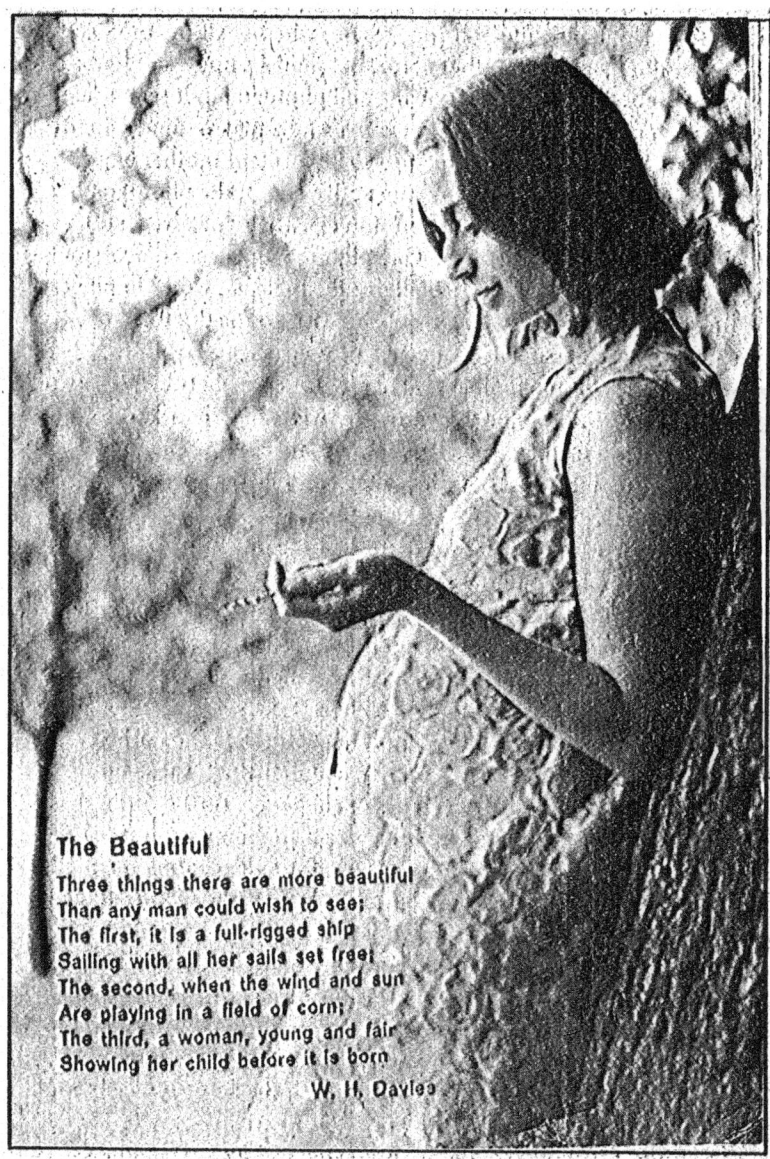

Fig. 2

in other photographic illustrations, where, whether sitting or standing, alone or with another actor, the model's body and limbs are typically unoccupied.[50] The drawing and photograph, it seems, are selectively employed to portray an active and a passive dimension to pregnancy. The graphic artist records the expectant mother engaged in the business of 'having a baby' (an active state); the photographer captures her simply 'being pregnant' (an essentially passive state). A finer distinction can be made. One picture sequences an occasion when the institutional, and particularly the medical, world impinges on pregnancy, in this instance, through a visit to the doctor. The other evokes the personal significance of pregnancy as captured in its more photogenic moments. These differences between the two types of illustration can be drawn out by widening the discussion from an analysis of these specific examples to a more general examination of the images of pregnancy contained in photographs and drawings.

Photographs of expectant mothers, like the one in Fig. 2, tend to employ special techniques — focus, close-up, cropping, lighting and angle — which together combine to create firstly, a *nucleus* and secondly, a *mood* for the photograph. The nucleus lies in the foreground and particularly in the pregnant woman, while the mood is one of tranquillity and other-worldliness. Focus, for example, is used to emphasise part of the picture, the actor, and fade other parts, the setting, which become misty and indistinct. Close-up and cropping (cutting off some parts of the body) further draw attention to the foreground and blur the surrounding landscape. Cropping, in addition, has another effect, for by excluding the model's legs, her abdomen becomes the central feature of the picture to which one's eyes are inevitably drawn. The use of lighting similarly draws attention to the actor, and to the contours of her body which stand out as if in silhouette against a contrasting backcloth. The outline of the body is emphasised more dramatically by the angle at which the photograph is taken. The model rarely stands facing the camera, a transverse view is much more popular, with the actor typically looking out to the right of the picture.

The sense of mood and emphasis created by these techniques is more explicitly developed in the content of the illustrations: in the setting, props and character of the actor. As regards *setting*, outdoor scenes are popular, with middle-class semi-detached interiors a second choice. Institutional and medical settings are scrupulously avoided, as are domestic scenes, the kitchen and bathroom. The few photographs set inside the house typically feature the sitting-room, where the mother is seen relaxing rather than busily engaged in household chores. In these pictures, symbols of health and nature are often included as props — for example, in one Lucozade advertisement, the model is placed beside a bowl of fruit, dreamily contemplating the suburban garden glimpsed through the french window of her sitting-room.[51] Similarly, the pages in the Mothercare catalogue devoted to maternity wear invariably provide their models with a range of naturalistic props — fruit, flowers, ferns. The partiality for the open air is restricted to certain kinds of setting, in particular to English summer landscapes of parks, greens and gardens. In these scenes — depicted for example in the illustration from *You and Your Baby* (Fig. 1), in the Health Education Council Leaflet, *When You are Pregnant*, and in a Cow and Gate baby milk advertisement, the sun is invariably shining and the picture full of summer-time symbols, green leaves, flowers, ducks, ice-cream.[52]

The similarity in setting is reflected in the composition of the female *actors*, whose likeness extends beyond their common anatomical condition. The models featured in photographs are apparently healthy and free from the debilitating side-effects associated with pregnancy. There is an homogeneity of age, race, height and implied social status, with certain categories of expectant mothers — the reproductively old, the short, the non-caucasoid, the overweight — excluded altogether. Hair, too, is standardised. Most models have long, free-flowing, loose hair with only a few pictured with short, set styles. The 'naturalness' of the hair is reflected in the clothes, which are typically of a soft, diaphanous material with long sleeves and a high, ruffled neck-line. Flowery prints and smocks are also popular but the heavy maternity wear of trousers and coats featured in maternity catalogues rarely appear. Marital status is usually spelt out, although recently, photographers have become less obsessed with this aspect of appearance. A few years ago, pictures were elaborately constructed to make marital status unambiguous, with the left hand displayed, however contrived it may look, in a prominent position on a chair or the abdomen.[53] Today, a male actor, young, white, dark-haired and casually dressed, is sometimes introduced as a substitute for a wedding ring. He, although making marital status somewhat equivocal, serves an additional function in conveying the symbolic marital significance of pregnancy.[54]

Where the model is not featured alone, the relationship between the actors is rarely of the reciprocal, two-way variety, with each the

centre of the other's attention. Instead, the photographs portray
either divergent relationships, with the expectant mother and her
co-actor directed towards something different, or more usually, a
semi-reciprocal relationship, where the supporting actor looks at
the pregnant woman, but she is looking elsewhere. The focus of her
attention in such photographs is interesting. It is not other objects
that absorb her attention — even when the object is the product being
advertised — nor is the reader the focus of attention. Instead, she is
staring into the middle distance, or less frequently at herself. In the
former case, although she may well be watching something out of view
of the camera, one gets the feeling that she isn't, in fact, looking at
anything in particular. While others demonstrate concern and
affection for her, she is lost in a state of reverie. The way in which
tactility is used underlines her emotional orientation. While the male
actor uses his arms to actively protect her, her body posture suggests
a self-orientation. Her hands are used to draw attention to and
embrace herself and particularly her abdomen and by implication,
her child. Similarly, in facial expression, with the slight smile and
distant eyes, it is possible to detect a narcissistic element, a feeling
of contented preoccupation.

Superimposing together these features of form and content
produces a finely drawn portrait of pregnancy.[55] Pregnancy, as seen
in photographs, is a personal affair. It is a time when a woman pays
attention to her body and her emotions rather than to other actors
and inanimate objects. The pregnant woman, unlike the mother after
birth, does not act upon her external world, but relaxes in it — or
escapes from it to another reality where, in a state of nature,
surrounded by sun and greenery, she discovers her femininity. She is
neither erotic nor exotic. Instead, although sexual involvement is
an unavoidable pre-requisite of pregnancy, she is portrayed as pure and
innocent — even to the extent of being clothed in white.

This idealised image of pregnancy stands in marked contrast to
the image contained in the drawings of pregnant women. In form,
drawings, like the one reproduced in Fig. 1, or those found in *You and
Your Baby*, lack the sophisticated techniques of cropping and close-up,
lighting and focus. In content, they are dull and functional compared
to their photographic counterparts. The *settings* are dominated not by
naturalistic outdoor scenes, but by functional interiors. Further, the
pictures feature not the domestic, front-room scenes popular in the
photographs, but rather the non-domestic institutional settings —
offices, doctors' surgeries, hospitals. Like settings, the choice of props

includes those omitted from the photographic repertoire. Props are invariably utilitarian — the stethoscope, pen and prescription pad in Fig. 1, the apples and milk jugs featured in *You and Your Baby* cartoons, the ubiquitous pillow in the illustrations of antenatal exercises.[56] Although utilitarian, such props are not without metaphorical value. For the props and the actors who employ them depict the preventive measures — medical supervision, diet, exercise — which are seen as necessary to a healthy pregnancy. Health, thus, appears not as something automatically ascribed to pregnancy (as in the photographs), but rather something individually achieved through diligence and obedience.

The characteristics of the *actors* bring out again this practical and prescriptive orientation. The homogeneity of photographic models as regards age, physique and social status is less noticeable and although some drawings attempt to delineate the long hair and soft features associated with femininity, most settle for an ageless, expressionless dummy dressed to suit the role she is illustrating — whether visiting the doctor, resting in bed, doing exercises or going to work. The floral smocks and dresses of the photographs are less in evidence, and trousers, excluded in photographs, are occasionally worn. Hair styles, too, tend to be more restrained and practical, with some models pictured with their hair cut and set in a way reminiscent of the fashion of the '50s (the *You and Your Baby* drawings of antenatal posture and relaxation for example).[57] The stance and pose of the models is no longer relaxed and reclining, with limbs arranged to caress and protect the body. Instead, the figures are stiff and lifeless, representing what one supposes is good posture in pregnancy, with limbs orientated to the practical matter in hand. Turning to the pattern of relationships between actors, we find that these are less elaborated than in photographs. Fewer pictures include other actors, and in those that do, the relationship tends to be of the more conventional reciprocal type, with each actor orientated to the other, as for example in the illustration of doctor-patient interaction (Fig. 1). Where there are no co-actors, the model's attention is typically object-orientated, to the glass of milk in the *You and Your Baby* cartoon, or activity-orientated, to doing her exercises, a pattern which again contrasts with the other-worldly, middle-distance gaze of the photographic model.[58]

Viewed as a whole, it seems that these features of form and content contain an image of pregnancy different from and in opposition to that portrayed in photographs. The graphic image and the photographic image of pregnancy diverge and conflict in three critical respects.

Firstly, the *nature* of being pregnant is differently perceived. In photographs, pregnancy appears as narcissistic and contemplative — and healthy. In drawings pregnancy is seen as physiological and practical, and the possibility of ill health, although not spelt out, can be inferred from non-performance of the antenatal routines that the cartoon figures demonstrate. Thus while in photographs we find the models absorbed in passive, psychological and essentially non-functional pursuits: in drawings, the dummies are engaged, but rarely absorbed, in active, physical and health-giving occupations, eating, drinking, doing their exercises. Even ostensibly contemplative activities, relaxing on the floor or in the chair, have a deliberate, functional orientation at odds with the other-wordly mood of the photographs. While the model in the photograph, contemplates herself, her child-in-utero and her future role, the cartoon dummy does something about these matters: she watches her diet, she rests and does exercises, she knits and shops, she visits her doctor. She interprets the meaning of her pregnancy in practical rather than symbolic terms.

Secondly, drawings and photographs portray the *control* of pregnancy in different ways. In photographs, activities, relationships and posture are generally self-selected and self-directed; in drawings they are chosen and directed by others. The models do their exercises, eat apples, drink milk, rest daily, and visit their doctor, not necessarily because they choose to, but because of a feeling of obligation. There is an implied duty made explicit in the text which accompanies the drawings, to one's doctor and to one's baby, an obligation that brings with it a sense that the activities depicted in the drawings are being watched and supervised by external observers.

Thirdly, in drawings and photographs pregnancy is set in a different *context*. Photographs place pregnancy in a world of personal relationships, where settings, props and actors combine to convey a sense of the femininity of the occasion: the beauty, the romance, the fulfilment. Drawings, by contrast, locate pregnancy in a world of impersonal and institutional relationships, where notions of femininity are noticeably absent. Instead, settings, props and actors are used to emphasise not her mystic and emotional qualities but rather her physiological role as the vehicle of reproduction. The expectant mother is transformed into an automated machine which must be regularly fed, exercised and overhauled, with the responsibility for her supervision and maintenance delegated to the medical profession.

This dualistic representation of pregnancy, with its contrasting image of nature, control and context, is similarly apparent in the texts which accompany the illustrations of expectant mothers. It seems to result, I suggest, from the incorporation of a narcissistic dimension into a predominantly physiological and medicalised model of childbearing. I have traced the origins of this ambivalent image by drawing out themes, about the importance of psychology *v.* physiology, about health *v.* sickness and self *v.* medical care, which appear as a historical dialogue in the development of antenatal literature. Like the previous pedagogies of pregnancy, the philosophies of health and hygiene which dominated nineteenth- and early twentieth-century literature, the contemporary image functions to support a particular style of antenatal care. In this model, the doctor appears to have surrendered a considerable portion of his power to the woman and her husband, who are granted a license to manage and enjoy the emotional and relational aspects of pregnancy. However, their authority is, in reality restricted to those peripheral and residual areas of maternity care in which medical personnel generally have little interest. The doctor maintains ultimate control over all matters relating to physiological management and thus over the vital questions of what is done to the woman's body, when it is done and how it is done. This demarcation of authority, intimated in the texts of popular guides, is made more explicit in the illustrations. It says, in effect, that a narcissistic and self-directed approach to pregnancy is conditional upon and secondary to the woman's acceptance of a higher medical prerogative. Photographs give us a glimpse of pregnancy as enjoyable, emotional and in harmony with nature; drawings reveal, behind this perspective, the reality of medicalised antenatal care.

Notes

1. The historical changes in attitudes to children and child care is covered by Phillippe Aries, *Centuries of Childhood* (New York, Knopf, 1962); William Kessen, *The Child* (London, John Wiley and Sons, 1968); Ivy Pinchbeck and Margaret Hewitt, *Children in English Society Vol. I and II* (London, Routledge and Kegan Paul, 1973). Contemporary patterns of child-rearing are described in John and Elizabeth Newson, *Patterns of Infant Care* (London, George Allen and Unwin, 1963), and *Four Years Old in an Infant Community* (London, George Allen and Unwin, 1968); Robert Sears, Eleoner Macoby and Harvey Levin, *Patterns of Childrearing* (London, Harper and Row, 1957); Margaret Mead and Martha Wolfenstein, *Childhood in Contemporary Cultures* (London, University of Chicago Press, 1955).
2. Martha Wolfenstein observes about the contemporary experts who offer

34 Health Care and Health Knowledge

information and guidance to parents: 'Those who mediate between science and the lay public often draw on their own and currently prevailing moral attitudes to derive practical recommendations. Thus child-training literature is as much expressive of the moral climate of the time in which it is written as the state of knowledge about children.' (Mead and Wolfenstein, 1955, p. 145.)

3. Examples of the definition of pregnancy as a 'natural process', and the subsequent qualifications of this definition can be found in most popular guides. Books include Gordon Bourne, *Pregnancy* (London, Pan, 1975), p. vii and *You and Your Baby, Part I* (Family Doctor Publications, 1975), p. 24. Examples in magazines can be found in Good Housekeeping Editorial Bulletin, 'Antenatal and post natal care', p. 1, and *Mother*, Jan. 1974, p. 34 ('Care in Pregnancy').
4. *You and Your Baby*, p. 43.
5. Bourne, p. 1.
6. *You and Your Baby*, pp. 21-2.
7. James H. Aveling, *English Midwives, Their History and Prospects* (London, Hugh Elliot Ltd., 1967); Harvey Graham, *Eternal Eve: The Mysteries of Birth and the Customs that surround it* (London. Hutchinson, 1960); James Ricci, *One Hundred Years of Gynaecology* (Philadelphia, The Blakiston Company, 1945).
8. Quoted in Harvey, 1960, op. cit.
9. Dr Hugh Chamberlen, *The Accomplisht Midwife*, 1673, quoted in Alice Clark, *Working Life of Women in the Seventeenth Century* (London, George Routledge and Sons, 1919).
10. Quoted in Aveling.
11. For example, see *Aristotle's Compleat and Experienced Midwife*, printed and sold by the booksellers, London, 1700; *The Works of Aristotle* (including *The Family Physician, The Experienced Midwife, the Book of Problems*), printed for the booksellers, London, 1796.
12. *The works of Aristotle*, 1850 edition, printed for the booksellers, London, by Mathieson and Co., p. 252.
13. Fleetwood Churchill, *Observations on the diseases incident to pregnancy and childbirth* (Dublin, Martin Keense and Sons, 1850), p. 4.
14. Samuel Ashwell, *A Practical Treatise on Parturition* (London, Thomas Tegg, 1828), p. 161.
15. Churchill, p. 14; William F. Montgomery, *An exposition of the signs and symptoms of pregnancy, the period of human gestation and the signs of delivery* (London, 1837), p. 12.
16. *The Works of Aristotle*, p. 215.
17. *The Works of Aristotle*, p. 216.
18. In addition to Graham and Ricco, referred to in 7 above, the nineteenth-century social assumptions concerning women's reproductive role and gynaecological processes are discussed in Martha Vicinus (ed.), *Suffer and Be Still: Women in the Victorian Age* (Bloomington, 1972); Mary Hartman and Lois Banner, *Cleo's Consciousness Raised: New Perspectives on the History of Women* (London, Harper Torchbooks, 1974); Patricia Branca, *Silent Sisterhood: Middle-Class Women in the Victorian Home* (London, Croom Helm, 1975). For an account of the personal experiences of child-bearing women see Women's Co-operative Guild, *Maternity: Letters from Working Women* (London, G. Bell and Sons, 1915).
19. The discussion of Victorian antenatal guides is based on the following books: Dr Pye Henry Chavasse, *Advice to a wife on the Management of her own health* (London, 1842); Dr Thomas Bull, *Hints to Mothers for the*

Management of Health During the Period of Pregnancy and in the Lying Room (London, Longmans, Orme, Brown, Green and Logmans, 1837); George Black, *The Young Wife's Advice Book, A guide for mothers on health and self management* (London, Ward, Lock and Co., 1880); Florence Stacpoole, *Advice to women on the care of their health before during and after confinement* (London, 1892); G. T. Wrench, *The Healthy Marriage* (London, J. and A. Churchill, 1911).

20. Stacpoole, p. 1.
21. Chavasse, p. 235.
22. Black, p. 20. In many ways, the attitudes to pregnant women, at the epitome of their femininity can be seen to exemplify attitudes to (upper-class) women in general. The notion of female frailty and vulnerability is discussed by the authors cited in reference 18.
23. For a discussion of the history of women's literature, see Cynthia White, *Women's Magazines, 1693-1968* (London, Michael Joseph, 1970).
24. John and Elizabeth Newsom see the control of the environmental and post-natal causes of infant mortality as crucial in the increasing orientation to child psychology. ('Cultural aspects of child rearing in the English speaking world', in Martin P. H. Richards, *The Integration of a Child into a Social World* (Cambridge University Press, 1974).) This also seems to have been a key factor in the emergence of the concept of antenatal care. The eugenic interest in the concept was made explicit by Lloyd George in 1911 (Birmingham Speech, 10 June 1911).

> The first thing we do in our (Insurance) bill is to provide adequate medical treatment for every workman in the kingdom. What next? We have a provision for maternity – an allowance of 30s. – money meant for the mother to help her in discharging her sacred function of motherhood by proper treatment and fair play, so as to put an end to this disgraceful infant mortality which we have got in this country.

25. Chavasse, p. 3.
26. Mabel Liddiard, *The Mothercraft Manual* 1928 edition, p. 10.
27. The increasing concern with the health of the poor can be linked to a range of factors, including the recognition of the demographic patterns of differential class fertility and the realisation of high morbidity levels among male working class in the aftermath of the Boer War. Such factors are discussed in the context of the changing child care principles at the turn of the century in Peter Wright, *The Birth of Child Rearing as a technical field and its importance as a form of social control*, paper presented at the British Sociological Association, 1976.
28. The antenatal movement was organised under the auspices of the National League for Maternal and Child Welfare. The League launched it through the Child Welfare Movement as an adjunct to their campaign for the establishment of Infant Welfare Centres. One of the first recorded antenatal schemes was introduced in Edinburgh in 1913, based initially on home visits but later extended through the establishment of an antenatal clinic. These early schemes were given legal sanction in the 1918 Maternity and Child Welfare Act. This act, which was permissive, not statutory, confirmed the local authorities' power to establish clinics, provide dental treatment, home visiting and educational classes for pregnant women. Reflecting the origins of the antenatal movement, antenatal care was organised as an extension of the child welfare department and not as part

36   *Health Care and Health Knowledge*

of the midwifery service. See G. F. McCleary, *The Maternity and Child Welfare Movements* (London, King. 1935). The Royal College of Obstetricians and Gynaecologists, *A National Maternity Service*, 1944.
29. Frederik Truby King, *Feeding and Care of Baby*, 1921, p. 153.
30. Science of Life, *Before and After Baby Comes*, 1958, p. 30, their italics.
31. Liddiard, p. 2.
32. Truby King, p. 99.
33. Ibid.
34. Truby King, *The Expectant Mother and Baby's First Month*, 1922.
35. Grantley Dick Read, *Natural Childbirth* (London, Heinemann, 1933).
36. Grantley Dick Read, *Childbirth Without Fear*, revised and edited by Helen Lessel, Harlan F. Ellis, 1972 (originally published 1944).
37. Dick Read, *Natural Childbirth*, chap. 5. He notes, for example, 'any emotional variations of the mother . . . may in some way affect the nutrition and metabolism of the unborn child'.
38. Ibid., p. 86.
39. J. Ransom, 'A brief history of British Methods of Antenatal Training during the first half of the century', in *Psychosomatic Medicine and Childbirth* (Paris, Ganthiers Villars, 1965).
40. Including Mary Barfield, *Relaxation for Childbirth* (London, Heinemann, 1960); Lee Buxton, *A Study of Psychophysical Methods for Relief of Childbirth* (Pan, Sanders, 1962); Helen Heardman, *The Way to Natural Childbirth* (Livingstone, 1964); Helen Heardman, *Relaxation and Exercises for Natural Childbirth* (Livingstone, 1964); Shiela Kitzinger, *The Experience of Childbirth* (Gollancz, 1962); Pierre Vellay, *Childbirth Without Pain* (Allen and Unwin, 1959); Erna Wright, *The New Childbirth* (Tandem, 1964).
41. *You and Your Baby*, first published 1957; *Having a Baby*, first published 1956; *Preparing to Have Your Baby*, 1964; *Letters to an Expectant Mother*, 1964.
42. Examples of the verbal acknowledgement, but de facto rejection of natural childbirth is found in many popular guides. A good instance is Alan Guttmacher, *Pregnancy and Birth* (Signet, 1962), in his description of a spontaneous birth (chap. 14, pp. 142-67). The way natural child birth is interpreted and distorted in hospitals is described in Nancy Stoller Shaw, *Forced Labor: Maternity Care in the United States* (Pergamon Press, 1974), and Suzanne Arms, *Immaculate Deception, A New Look at Women and Childbirth in America* (San Francisco Book Company, 1975).
43. The realities of antenatal care, and the ways it underlines the achievement of a natural, self-directed childbirth is described by Stoller Shaw.
44. The early sixties witnessed the success of a number of films in the popular cinema which revolved around or featured aspects of the child-bearing process. These included *A Taste Of Honey*, *The L-Shaped Room*, *Poor Cow* and *Rosemary's Baby*.
45. See reference 38.
46. In *Mother and Baby*, for example, the first illustration of a visibly pregnant woman appeared in 1964, although maternity fashions, using slim models, had been a regular feature in the magazine since it was first launched in 1956. It was not until the early '70s that the use of the 'bulge' became commonplace. Caution was clearly necessary in this area, as the experiences of *Women's Mirror*, who featured a colour front-page of a child-in-utero in 1965, indicates. (See Cynthia White for the full story.)
47. Trevor Millum, *Images of Women, Advertising in Women's Magazines* (London, Chatto, 1975).

48. *You and Your New Baby* is prepared by the Department of Health and Social Security and the Central Office of Information (1973); *You and Your Baby: Part I, Pregnancy and Birth* is produced by the British Medical Association (1973 edition). Family Doctor publications distribute 750,000 copies of *You and Your Baby* annually and claim that 90 per cent of pregnant women receive a copy.
49. For example, *You and Your Baby* (1970), pp. 26, 27, 43, 44, 46; 1973, pp. 38-9; 1975, p. 51; Expectant Mother Services, *Having a Baby* (1975), pp. 13 and 15.
50. Good examples are found on the covers of such antenatal literature as: *You and Your Baby*, 1970, 1973, 1975; Laurence Pernoud, *Nine Months to Motherhood* (London, 1975); Gordon Bourne, *Pregnancy* (Pan, 1975); as well as on the inside pages: for example, *You and Your Baby* (1975), pp. 11, 15, 23, 25.
51. Featured in *Mother and Baby* in 1973/4. Other examples of the use of naturalistic symbols in interior settings can be found in the sources cited above (reference 50).
52. Health Education Council, *When You Are Pregnant* (L22); the Cow and Gate baby milk advertisement, showing an expectant mother (long-haired, young, Caucasian and dressed in white) staring across a lake, appeared in *Mother and Baby* in 1973 and 1974.
53. For example, *You and Your Baby* (1970), cover picture and photographs on pp. 7 and 38; *You and Your Baby* (1973), pp. 20, 44, 56.
54. *You and Your Baby* (1973 and 1975), contain four photographs in their texts in which a man accompanies the pregnant model. In the 1970 edition there were none.
55. Some photographs deviate from this characteristic. For example, the photograph of pregnant women doing their exercises in the Health Visitors' Association publication, *New Baby* (1973), p. 11, fails to conform to the model in almost every respect and its realistic depiction creates almost a caricature of the image displayed in other photographs. An emergent realism is apparent in other new publications: see the photograph of mothers buying baby clothes in the 1975 edition of *You and Your Baby*.
56. The annual editions of *You and Your Baby*, the various Family Doctor publications on pregnancy (*Having A Baby, Preparing to Have Your Baby, You and Your Pregnancy*) and Expectant Mother Services, *Having a Baby* (1975), provide the best examples of the techniques employed in drawings: institutional settings, utilitarian props, 'dummy' models, reciprocal relationships between actors.
57. *You and Your Baby* (1970), pp. 51-3; (1973), pp. 38-9; (1975), pp. 49-51.
58. The cartoons of the expectant mother with glass of milk and apple in hand appear in *You and Your Baby* (1970), pp. 26 and 27.

Sally Macintyre, in the paper which follows, shows not only that old age has not always been seen as a problem but that the kind of problem it is seen to be has varied over time. Before the 1890s the old were seen simply as part of the larger category of infirm or able-bodied destitute, age itself did not constitute a social problem. Since that date old age has been singled out as problematic, but the emphasis has varied. In some periods in the decades around the turn of the century for example, the stress has been on reducing the suffering entailed for the old people themselves. In other periods, notably in the 1940s, stress has been on the cost to the society as a whole of maintaining the old who do not, and never again will, contribute to production.

Macintyre, following Waller, shows that these two approaches are inevitably in tension: to improve the standard of life and the services available to the elderly is to reduce resources available for other categories in society. Macintyre convinces us that the apparent solution to this dilemma, which it was thought had been found in the fifties and early sixties, was in fact a mirage. It was then believed that active medical treatment, along with domiciliary care, would at one and the same time reduce the cost of caring for the elderly *and* improve their life circumstances. But emptying the residential institutions was pursued more vigorously than was providing care in localities and the costs of providing domiciliary care were never carefully computed. If in fact cheaper than residential care, domiciliary care may well only be so because of the unpaid labour of families, neighbours and volunteers (all including a majority of women, one might add). Nor were the wishes of the old people themselves ever taken into account and indeed, as Macintyre points out, while not impossible this is difficult to do. Certainly, there is evidence that some at least, among both rich and poor, opt for residential care rather than independence or life with a family. The quality of care depends much on relative affluence and there is a sense in which old age is only a problem to the aged when it is associated with poverty.

Macintyre believes that the conflict between the welfare of the old (the humanitarian perspective) and the burden on the rest of society (the organisational perspective) cannot be resolved. She wisely warns that any policy for the elderly should be looked at critically with a recognition of the presence of this conflict in mind. She suggests that demographic changes cannot account for fluctuations in attention to old age or the content of the policies. She hints towards the end of her review that times of national economic hardship, like the present, may tend to the organisational perspective, however well disguised with humanitarian rhetoric. She does not develop this argument, however; nor does she set the changes she records in perspectives in their historical periods with their social and economic contexts. But that was not her aim. Why did welfare predominate in the 1890s and 1920s? Why did the forties take an organisational perspective? One hopes that these questions will be answered in a later paper.

What is clear is that the conflict to which Macintyre refers is one which is found throughout the health and welfare sector. It is also one which derives from the prevailing social and economic organisation of society and from its associated values. In a society which values competition and achievement highly, where those who can contribute productive labour are rewarded and those who cannot are disvalued, how is one to ensure adequate humane care for the permanently unproductive? What is also clear from Macintyre's account is that even apparently humane medical policies can themselves be trapped within this conflict. The active treatment policy was justified on utilitarian grounds, although on balance its utility in terms of saving resources for society as a whole has, as Macintyre demonstrates, to be questioned. Another conflict is also present. The policy was humanely designed to reduce suffering, although at the same time it was designed to increase the demand for, and the status of, a medical specialty. Active treatment of the elderly was a medical policy which, because it could not have the socioeconomic consequences claimed for it, could never be fully implemented on socioeconomic grounds.

M.S.

OLD AGE AS A SOCIAL PROBLEM
Historical Notes on the English Experience

Sally Macintyre

Introduction

In this paper I examine changes in central government policies towards old age in England between 1834 and 1976. The paper is based on documents published by government departments and by commissions and committees of enquiry over this period. My main focus is on the *contents* of formulations of old age as a social problem, and upon their possible consequences. I argue that competing formulations of old age as a social problem produce certain tensions and dilemmas for the provision of medical and social services, and that these dilemmas may be equally relevant to other conditions and may currently be assuming increasing significance.

It is perhaps necessary here to point to those topics which I do not attempt to cover in this paper. I do not attempt to provide a comprehensive historical examination of the various policies and assumptions here described. Neither do I discuss the detailed implementation of them at a local level. Further, the policies described here refer only to England, and not, for example, to Scotland, which has experienced a different pattern of policies. These topics are not excluded because I regard them as unimportant or uninteresting. To explain the genesis of social policies, to describe their implementation, and to compare them across countries is an enormous task. I have therefore chosen here to address a more limited set of questions about the assumptions and implications of certain social policies. In the space available, attempting to do more might involve glossing over some of the more interesting features of these policies.

Old Age as a Social Problem

Fuller and Myers have suggested that 'Social problems are what people think they are, and if conditions are not defined as social problems by the people involved in them, they are not problems to those people, although they may be problems to outsiders or to scientists.' (1941, p. 320.) They have further suggested that every social problem consists of two components, an objective condition and a subjective definition, and described the former as being necessary but not sufficient to produce the latter. Blumer (1971) has laid greater stress on the subjective definition, suggesting that the objective condition is of secondary importance, while Becker (1966) and Lemert (1951) have gone even further in suggesting that the objective existence of a condition is not even necessary for the subjective definition, i.e. that persons can define non-existent conditions as social problems. Following the perspective used by such writers, I use the words 'problem' or 'social problem' in this paper as meaning 'problems as perceived by persons in the society'.

It has often been suggested that the definition of any condition as a social problem may involve formally similar processes, and a number of different models of the 'natural history of a social problem' have been outlined.[1] Interest in such natural histories focuses attention on the *form* of problem definition, and in so doing may divert attention from the *content* of the definitions. I would argue that the contents of such definitions may be crucial in that they provide, implicitly or explicitly, recipes for remedial action. As Becker notes: 'Arguments over measures to be taken are often difficult to resolve precisely because the varying answers to the questions are contained, waiting to be deduced, in the definitions proposed by supporters of different measures.' (1966, p. 10.)

The content of definitions of social problems, and their implications for action, have usually been studied in terms of differences between groups with conflicting interests.[2] Any one group or individual may, however, have a number of different interests whose coexistence may produce contradictory and conflicting definitions and recipes for action. Waller has suggested that all social problems exist within a moral universe, and because of this are characterised by competing interests:

> A simple formulation of our standpoint, which we advocate as roughly accurate for most social problems, rests upon the assumption of two conflicting sets of mores. Social problems result from the interaction of these two groups of mores, which we may call the organisational and humanitarian mores . . . Value judgements are the formal causes of social problems, just as the law is the formal cause of crime . . . The same mores from which the deplored conditions arise continue to operate to limit any action which one takes in order to remedy them. (1936: 1971 edition, pp. 96, 97.)

Conflicts may arise not only between different groups in their formulations of social problems, but also between the organisational

Old Age as a Social Problem

and humanitarian mores of any one person or group. Policies premised on either organisational or humanitarian mores may conflict with one another. Further, over time there may be changes in the stress given to either the organisational or humanitarian interests at the expense of the other. It is to this tension between conflicting interests that this paper is addressed.

The above general points can now be applied specifically to old age. Firstly, the amount of concern expressed about old age, and whether it has been perceived to be socially problematic by policy makers and administrators, has varied considerably in England. In some periods an interest in old age has been fashionable and in other periods it has virtually been ignored. Up until the 1890s there is no evidence of old age having been singled out as a discrete social problem meriting particular attention. Between 1890 and 1910, however, there was a considerable outpouring of concern for, and attention to, old age as evinced in a number of government reports and enquiries.[3]

This interest then died down after about 1910 and was replaced by concern about other social problems. It was revived in the 1940s and 1950s, with the 'problem of old age' being a major concern of the reconstruction period.[4] This concern was muted in the mid-1960s, attention then being focused on other problems such as education and child poverty. Similarly, the spate of books and articles on social gerontology and old age which appeared in the 1950s and early 1960s dried up in the late 1960s.[5] There is some evidence, however, that in the last year or so there has been yet another resurgence of interest.[6]

Secondly, these changes in the fashionableness of old age as a topic of concern do not appear to be attributable solely to empirical changes in the number or condition of the elderly, but rather to changes in perceptions of their numbers and condition. For example, the Majority Report of the 1909 Royal Commission noted that while it had received considerable evidence from individuals to the effect that the proportion of the elderly on poor relief was increasing, there had been a *decrease* in the rate of aged pauperism to population since 1870 (1909; para 344).[7]

The concern in the 1940s sprang from a perception of a declining birth-rate and increased longevity which, taken together, would increase the proportion of the elderly in the population. The 'numbers problem' remained in existence during the 1960s and the decline in interest cannot be attributed solely to a better-than-expected set of demographic figures. It may instead be attributable to differing perceptions of the key problems of the day. For example, the 're-discovery' of poverty in Britain and the USA (Abel Smith and Townsend, 1965; Harrington, 1963) shifted attention from the so-called problems of affluence, including old age, back to problems of scarcity. No longer did one see books like Bernard's *Social Problems at Mid-Century: Role, Status and Stress in a Context of Abundance* (1957) in which it was argued that all the problems of scarcity had been solved and that new, psychological problems had emerged within a context of abundance. Attention was re-directed towards family poverty, single parent families, and the conservation of resources.[8] There is no evidence that these changing concerns were simple responses to the stimuli of objective changes in the population or in the incidence or magnitude of family poverty. Similarly, there is no evidence that the recent resurgence in interest can be attributed to demographic changes (particularly since when it started it coexisted with a continuing concern to reduce the birthrate) or to radically changed health and social conditions among the aged.

Thirdly, there have not only been changes in whether old age is considered to be a social problem; there have also been changes in what sort of problem it has been considered to be, and in the remedies seen as appropriate to solve these problems. The concerns expressed at the turn of the century were very different from those expressed in the 1940s, which differed again from those expressed in the 1960s.

It is possible to isolate two different formulations of old age as a social problem. Firstly, there is what, following Waller (1936), I shall describe as a humanitarian perspective. From this stance old age is viewed as problematic because it entails suffering and costs for individual old people − poverty, ill health, incapacity, loneliness, lack of prestige and dignity, etc. In terms of action, such a formulation involves consideration of how best to ameliorate or prevent these problems associated with the aging process by reducing the individual costs of aging to the old person.

Secondly, there is what, also following Waller, I shall describe as the organisational perspective. From this stance, old age is formulated as being a social problem because of the burden of dependency it places on society as a whole, or on the productive members of society. In terms of action such a formulation involves consideration of how best to reduce the social costs imposed on the community by the elderly population.

At the extreme, the humanitarian solution to the perceived problems of old age is a massive redistribution of resources, power and prestige from younger age groups to the elderly; the organisational solution to the perceived problems of old age would be something like the Eskimo one — euthanasia or suicide on the day of retirement from productive life. The first solution would involve, among other things, a reductuon in the GNP, problems in the balance of payments, diversion of resources from children and adults who might have been able to provide some productive return for that investment, and changes in the promotion chances of the young, all of which conflict with organisational interests. The second solution would clearly conflict with humanitarian values.

Old age may thus be viewed as similar to other forms of permanent incapacity, and dissimilar to other conditions such as childhood or acute illness in adults, in that the two perspectives — humanitarian and organisational — are potentially in conflict with one another. Education may be seen as beneficial both as enhancing the fulfilment of individuals and as constituting investment in human capital; services for mothers and young children as beneficial in terms of both individual health and happiness and as ensuring the productive or fighting capacity of the next generation; and the treatment of acute illness episodes in working adults as being a citizen's right as well as a useful means of expeditiously returning people to the work force. Provision for the elderly has rarely, however, been seen to have such dual pay-offs: not only may it be viewed as having no positive investment functions, it may also be seen as producing negative returns on investment by keeping persons alive and consuming resources even longer than they would have done without that care.

In the remainder of this paper I examine the relative weight that at various times has been placed on the humanitarian and organisational perspectives, and examine post-war attempts to combine the two perspectives by the advocacy of 'community care'.

Humanitarian and Organisational Themes in Official Policy Towards Old Age

In this section I amplify and illustrate the points made above with reference to official documents from 1834 onwards. This period can be divided into five distinct periods each exemplifying different approaches to the problem of old age.

1834-1890

Most commentators agree that prior to 1890 old age was not distinguished as being a specific social problem meriting particular attention. Under both the Elizabethan and New Poor Law of 1834 the elderly infirm were regarded as but one sub-segment of the general category of 'impotent poor', and the elderly able-bodied poor as but one sub-segment of the general category of able-bodied destitute. Old age *per se* was not regarded as problematic, destitution or infirmity at any age being the criterion for relief. The Majority Report of the 1909 Royal Commission of the Poor Laws noted:

> The practice of considering the aged as a class by themselves for purposes of relief is one of modern growth. Throughout the history of the Poor Law we find old age regarded as one form of impotency; the distinction lay between the poor and impotent, on the one hand, and the able-bodied on the other. Sometimes the impotent and aged are mentioned together, but always as forming one class to be dealt with in one and the same way. (Part IV, para.304.)

The Royal Commission on the Poor Laws of 1832-4 had recommended that the deterrent principles of less eligibility should not be applied to the impotent poor. However, the policy established by the Poor Law Commissioners between 1834-47, and continued by the Poor Law Board of 1847-71, was one of 'indiscriminate use of the General Mixed Workhouse, tempered in practice by general outdoor relief to all kinds of aged and infirm' (Minority Report of the Royal Commission 1909, p. 906). The retention of the general mixed workhouse led to the application of the 'self-acting test' of less eligibility to the aged and infirm as well as to the able-bodied, while according to the 1909 Minority Report the outdoor relief given was 'indiscriminate, insufficient and unconditional' (p. 901).

Between 1871 and 1890 the 'test of the workhouse' was specifically advocated for the infirm and aged, as well as for the able-bodied, by the school of strict administrators epitomised by Sir Henry Longley at the Local Government Board. Longley suggested that such a deterrent policy would encourage people to save for their old age and infirmity, voluntary charity to support the 'deserving' infirm in order to protect them from the rigours and stigma of the workhouse, and relatives to support infirm individuals rather than see them in the workhouse:

Old Age as a Social Problem

It is, I believe, within the experience of many Boards of Guardians, that while there are persons who, even when in prosperous circumstances, readily permit their aged relations to receive out-relief, an offer of indoor relief is frequently found to put pressure upon them to rescue themselves, if not their relations, from the discredit incident to the residence of the latter in a workhouse. (Report on the Administration of Outdoor Relief in the Metropolis: 3rd Annual Report of the Local Government Board, 1873-74.)

Those Unions which implemented this deterrent policy in respect of the elderly and infirm were held up for admiration and approval by the Inspectors, and in Official Reports (Minority Report of the Royal Commission, 1909, p. 902).

Thus, between 1834 and 1890 the organisational concerns of the 1832-4 Royal Commission on the Poor Laws, i.e. the stress on reducing the burden of the Poor Rates by the principle of less eligibility, were directed to the elderly as constituting part of the larger categories of infirm or able-bodied destitute, initially by default (1834-71) and latterly as a matter of conscious principle (1871-90), by the administrators of the Poor Law. The major emphasis was with the interests of contributors to the Poor Rates rather than with the needs or desires of the beneficiaries.

1890-1910

However, during a twenty-year period from 1890 old age was singled out as constituting a discrete social problem, rather than as forming an occasional basis for inclusion in socially problematic classes such as the impotent poor, and as posing problems for the elderly themselves.

In official policy towards the implementation of the Poor Laws age *per se* began to be taken as a criterion for the granting of relief, and of relief of a different nature to that granted to other paupers. With official approval some parishes or unions set up scales of outdoor relief varying according to age.[9] Circulars issued by the Local Government Board in 1895 and 1896 laid down principles of workhouse administration for the elderly in complete contrast to those set out by Longley two decades earlier. The elderly were to be given a better diet, tobacco, more privacy in their sleeping arrangements, better physical facilities, and allowed to receive visitors and pay visits themselves. Committees visiting workhouses were enjoined to see that the aged were specially attended to, and to discuss any grievances with them in the absence of local officials. The Royal Commission on the Aged Poor (1895) endorsed proposals for the improvement of facilities for indoor relief for the elderly and recommended the provision of adequate outdoor relief, suggesting further that 'Such rules should be generally made known for the information of the poor of the Union, in order that those really in need may not be discouraged from applying.' (Quoted in Minority Report of the 1909 Royal Commission, p. 905.)

The focus within the administration of the Poor Law therefore shifted from one on a reduction in the number of persons in receipt of relief, and on the cost of providing such relief, to one of ensuring that all those in need obtained relief, and that the relief was adequate far above the level of subsistence.

As noted previously (see note 3) several Royal Commissions and select committees were set up to examine various aspects of the problems faced by the elderly. While the subject of the social costs of increased provision for the elderly was not ignored, the dominant theme was the humanitarian one of enhancing the welfare and happiness of old people.

For example, the Majority Report of the Royal Commission on the Poor Laws and Relief of Distress recommended that greater care should be taken to ensure 'adequacy of relief' for the elderly, and suggested that if they were unable to sustain an independent existence they should be provided with decent residential accommodation, preferably apart from the workhouse in small homes where they could keep their own possessions. It devoted attention to old persons who would benefit from residential care but who were not in receipt of it, and to morale and the retention of dignity within institutions. The proposed system of classifying the elderly in institutions by moral character was expounded in terms of the feelings of the respectable elderly, rather than in terms of the ratepayers' feelings.[10]

The Minority Report of the Royal Commission similarly emphasised the plight of elderly persons who needed residential care but who were not receiving it because of the harshness of the workhouse and its stigma of pauperism. In this sense it concentrated on the problems that the Poor Laws posed for elderly individuals, rather than vice versa, and its recommendations reflected this focus by stressing the need to get the elderly into institutions rather than out of them:

> By the staff of Health Visitors and Sanitary Inspectors, daily going their rounds, the Public Health Authority will become aware

Old Age as a Social Problem 49

of cases in which the helpless deserving aged, notwithstanding their little pensions or the attentions of the charitable, are suffering from neglect or lack of care. There ought, moreover, to be some practicable method by which a helpless old person may escape from or protect himself against the tyranny and repeated petty cruelties to which the aged are sometimes subjected, even by their own children. There should be for all such cases, available in every district, asylums or 'retreats under a more accurate and less degrading title' than that of the workhouse 'and under less stringent and kinder disciplines' . . . (1909, p. 922).

The other reports of the period similarly stressed the humanitarian perspective, e.g. the report of the Committee on Old Age Pensions commented:

Of the questions raised by the proposal to establish a State-aided pension system, that of its costs and administration is not the most serious. We do not question that the State could bear the necessary additional burden if the welfare of the community really demanded it. But would . . . it not affect the question of wages, and hand over to the employer rather than to the employed the benefit of the State contribution? Would the receipt of State aid be free from that taint of pauperism which makes Poor Law Relief bitter to the self-respect and independence of the best of the working classes? (1898, pp. 14-15.)

During this twenty-year period, in summary, old age was for the first time singled out as a social problem of concern to policymakers and administrators. The dominant theme within the official documents of the period was what I am here calling the humanitarian one, i.e. a perception of old age as bringing problems of various kinds to individuals, problems which the community should attempt to ameliorate through increased provision.[11]

The 1940s

During and immediately after the Second World War there was a revival of interest in old age as a social problem, but with rather a different focus from that expressed at the turn of the century. The official documents of the 1940s expressed concern about the burden of dependency produced by an increasing proportion of the elderly in the population.

Thus in his 1942 report, Beveridge started from what he called a diagnosis of want, based on the results of various pre-war surveys, and

> ... two other facts about the British community ... The first of these two facts is the age constitution of the population, making it certain that persons past the age that is now regarded as the end of working life will be a much larger proportion of the whole community than at any time in the past. The second fact is the low reproduction rate of the British community today ... The first fact makes it necessary to seek ways of postponing the age of retirement rather than hastening it. The second fact makes it imperative to give first place in social expenditure to the care of childhood and to the safe-guarding of maternity. (1942, para. 15.)

In referring to the elderly, the Beveridge report continually emphasised the problem of creating a balance between organisational and humanitarian interests, e.g.:

> The problem for the future is how persons who are past work can be given a guarantee against want in a form which gives the maximum of encouragement for voluntary saving for maintenance of standards above the subsistence minimum, and at the same time avoids spending money which is urgently needed elsewhere or money on a scale throwing an intolerable financial burden on the community. (1942, para. 238.)

and

> On the one hand, the provision made for age must be satisfactory; otherwise great numbers may suffer. On the other hand, every shilling added to pension rates is extremely costly in total ... It is dangerous to be in any way lavish to old age, until adequate provision has been assured for all other needs, such as the prevention of disease and the adequate nutrition of the young. (Para. 236.)

Thus, old age was formulated as a social problem because a commitment to meet the minimum needs of the elderly constituted a one-way drain on resources and a diversion of resources from other, more

Old Age as a Social Problem

pressing, areas of social need.

The 1949 Royal Commission on Population went even further than Beveridge in viewing old age as problematic from an organisational perspective. It defined the main problem of old age as being 'the fact that . . . the old consume without producing, which differentiates them from the active population and makes of them a factor reducing the average standard of living in the community' (para. 296). In its recommendations, it therefore concentrated on ways of reducing the social costs of old age, for example, suggesting that the old 'should, if possible, do more than hitherto to maintain themselves or rather contribute more by their exertions to the economic effort of the community' (para. 299).

It also presented an explicit plea to policy makers not to bend too far in the humanitarian direction:

> As the proportion of the electorate on pension is going to rise steadily, the strength of the pensioners as a political pressure group, already very considerable, may be expected to grow. Considerable political courage may therefore be needed to resist pressure for higher rates of benefit. It is most important that Ministers, Members of Parliament and public opinion at large should appreciate the implications of proposals to raise pension rates not only for the present but also for the future. (Para. 305.)

I am not arguing that the humanitarian perspective was entirely lacking in this literature of the 1940s, just as I do not argue that the organisational perspective was entirely lacking at the turn of the century. Rather, I am describing a shift in the relative emphasis placed on the two perspectives, and a differing view of the major problems created by old age. The emphasis on the social costs of old age in the two reports cited above may, for example, have been related to an assumption that the individual costs of old age had been reduced by the health and welfare measures of the period, and that the needs of the elderly were being adequately met by such provisions, leaving official concern free to devote itself to the problem of the social costs of such measures. Whatever the reasons, the literature of this period exemplifies, in almost ideal-typical form, concern with old age as a burden on the community.

The 1950s and 1960s

At the 1950 General Election the Labour Party declared that it had 'ensured full employment and fair shares of the necessities of life' and that 'destitution had been banished' (quoted in Bull, 1971, p. 13). However, during the early 1950s any such complacency about provision for the elderly was undermined in a series of official reports. An enquiry by the Ministry of Pensions and National Insurance showed that 54 per cent of the men who chose to stay at work after 65 did so for financial reasons (1954, para. 79), and the Phillips Report showed that a substantial number of old people lived on or near the borderline of poverty (1954, para. 109). The Boucher Report suggested that many elderly patients in hospital could have been discharged had they had adequate amenities and support in their own homes (1957).

Evidence that the provisions of the welfare state did not adequately meet all the perceived needs of the elderly coexisted with a continuing concern with the social costs of the welfare state. While in 1948 the Ministry of Health encouraged the construction of 'more humane' homes for the elderly, catering for 30-35 residents, by 1953 it was criticising local authorities for 'extravagance' in the design of homes, and by 1955 was suggesting that it might be more economical to build homes for up to 60 residents with multi-bedded rooms and smaller sitting rooms (Parker, 1962, pp. 109-10). The Guillebaud Committee, set up to review the costs of the National Health Service, noted that the demands made on the NHS by the elderly were increasing and attributed this increase both to the growing proportion of the elderly in the population and to an improvement in the quality of local authority and hospital accommodation which had stimulated demand (1956, para. 641).

Policy makers therefore saw themselves faced with an increasing burden placed on the health and welfare services by the elderly, and with evidence that the needs of the elderly were not being met, i.e. that both the organisational and humanitarian problems were persisting in tandem. One perceived solution to this problem — community care — was first explicitly proposed by the Phillips Report of 1954. In order to place this proposal in its context I shall digress briefly outside the sphere of central government policy.

During the 1940s certain clinicians began to see old age as a distinct field for medical attention, and became dissatisfied with the treatment currently given to the elderly — treatment that had evolved partially by default from the concentration given to acute illness episodes in younger persons. The Medical Society for the Care of the Aged was founded in 1947, partly as a forum for the discussion of these new ideas, and partly as a 'ginger group' to stimulate changes (Felstein, 1969). The new self-styled geriatricians proposed a dynamic and curative approach to the diseases of old age, aimed at rehabilitation to an active life in the community, to replace the 'tender loving care' that had been provided by their predecessors in chronic wards, and this approach was implemented at several hospitals.[12] It met, according to Felstein, with 'heavy opposition from hospital colleagues in the medical wards, who could not see the value of spending time, money, energy or bed space on redundant senior members of the community' (1969, p. 15). However, the success of this rehabilitative policy as measured in the high rate of turnover persuaded the Ministry of Health and Regional Hospital Boards of the feasibility of the approach, and money was gradually made available for the conversion of long-stay wards into rehabiliation units, and for the construction of purpose-built geriatric units, day hospitals, and outpatient clinics.

The development of the specialty of geriatrics was in some ways analogous to the development of paediatrics in the inter-war years, in that attention was focused on the elderly as a group exhibiting particular disease patterns to which principles derived from general adult medicine or surgery were not applicable. In another sense, however, the development of geriatrics brought the treatment of the elderly *closer* to the principles of adult medicine. The rehabilitative approach was based on assumptions taken from general medicine and surgery, namely that the aim of treatment and care was to return the individual to some normal, active, and self-supporting existence. Thus, in one way it underlined the differences between geriatric and adult medicine — instead of geriatricians providing maintenance functions in chronic wards, they were to adopt the curative and rehabilitative approach previously directed only to younger age groups, and the same standards of the 'good life' as were espoused for those age groups.

This rehabilitative approach was noted with approval by the Phillips Committee: 'This is a development which we welcome, both for the improvement it promises in health and happiness and for the relief to the heavy cost of looking after large numbers of chronic sick. Moreover, active younger people now employed in looking after them can now be released for other work.' (1954, para. 271.) Whereas Beveridge and the Royal Commission on Population had described services for the elderly as involving heavy social costs with only individual benefits, the Phillips Committee pointed out that the rehabilitative approach could be regarded as a short-term investment that would reduce later social costs: 'Adequate domiciliary services are essential if this policy is to be successful, and expenditure on these can often prevent greater cost and suffering later on . . .' (1954, para. 323). The report's key points were that (a) active medical treatment followed by domiciliary care in the community was cheaper than either long-stay hospital or residential care; (b) that the elderly much preferred to live independent lives in their own homes.

In the light of the difficulties of balancing organisational and individual interests as perceived in the previous decade, it is understandable why this approach was so attractive to policy makers and administrators. Having previously assumed that the incapacities of old age were irremediable, so creating an ever-increasing burden of care, here was evidence from the experiments of geriatricians that such incapacities were in many cases remediable and/or preventable, and that it was no longer necessary to assume that there was an inevitable process of decline in individual old people's capacity for self-care. By taking it as axiomatic that individual old people would prefer to be active, productive and independent, the Phillips Committee was able to present the concept of community care as being deeply humanitarian as well as organisationally efficient.

These assumptions made by the Phillips Committee became incorporated into official conventional wisdom, and were repeated throughout the decade in subsequent reports and proposals. For example, the Guillebaud Committee stated:

> The first aim should be to make adequate provision wherever possible for the treatment and care of old people in their own homes. The development of the domiciliary services for this purpose will be a genuine economy measure, and also a humanitarian measure in enabling old people to lead the sort of life they much prefer. (1956, para. 647.)

This policy was echoed in the building notes from the Ministry of Health, and in the early 1960s by the ten-year Hospital Plan which recommended a reduction in the ratio of geriatric beds to 10 per 1,000 elderly population, stating that 'With the further development of active treatment and rehabilitation and the wider and fuller provision for the elderly outside hospital, this ratio should be adequate or more than adequate . . .' (1962, para. 16).[13]

Old Age as a Social Problem

The work of social and medical scientists, among whom there was a marked 'anti-institution' fashion during this period, were cited in official reports as confirming these assumptions (e.g. Townsend, 1964; Barton, 1959; Bowlby, 1951). In the mental health field there was a parallel governmental emphasis on de-institutionalisation implemented in the 1959 Mental Health Act. All this was a far cry from the opposite concern expressed by both reports of the 1909 Royal Commission; namely, that old people who needed it were not obtaining residential care. All the emphasis was the other way round — the 'misplacement' of persons in hospitals and homes who should not have been there.

While all the official publications in the 1950s and 1960s mentioned the need to improve domiciliary services to cope with the increasing proportion of the elderly to be discharged from institutions, more space was devoted to proposals for reducing institutional provision than to proposals for increasing domiciliary provision. While the 1962 Hospital Plan constituted detailed proposals for a reduction of geriatric beds, the 1963 report, 'Health and Welfare: the Development of Community Care', contained only a summary of the plans drawn up by local authorities, with an explicit repudiation of any intention to issue detailed directives, e.g.: 'The purpose is therefore neither to lay down a standard pattern nor to state principles and objectives dogmatically.' (1963, p. iii.)

It could, of course, be argued that the division of administrative responsibilities meant that the central government only had power to influence the hospital sector, and that lack of attention in central government documents to domiciliary services simply reflected this powerlessness. However, even with regard to services over which it did have some authority, the central government showed some lack of interest. Under the permissive powers of the 1946 National Assistance Act all local authorities in England and Wales had introduced home help services, and by 1963, 75 per cent of cases attended were over 65. Local authorities pressed the central government for more home helps but were informed that inadequate finance precluded this. Chiropody services were not sanctioned until 1959, despite frequent appeals from local government; the provision of home meals was not sanctioned until 1962, and had to be introduced as a private member's bill. Section 13 of the 1968 Health Services and Public Health Act made home help services a statutory obligation, and empowered the provision of laundry facilities; it was not only considered long overdue by many local authority workers in the field but was immediately postponed. Financial priorities did not appear to bear out the policy of improving community services -- plans for spending £500 million in ten years on hospitals were not mirrored by any concrete plans for a concomitant increase in expenditure on domiciliary provision, while the organisational concerns were matched by plans for a reduction in institutional services relative to the population of the elderly.[14]

The assumptions of the Phillips Report were occasionally questioned. For example, the National Corporation for Old People showed in the mid-50s that the cost of providing domiciliary services was not necessarily less, in terms of manpower and money, and might in some cases be considerably more, than the cost of providing institutional care.[15] Similarly, Shenfield (1957) stressed that whether or not domiciliary services were cheaper than institutional ones depended on the amount of care given, and criticised the dictum that attempts should always be made to keep the elderly in their own homes. Official reports all continued, however, to treat it as axiomatic that domiciliary care was cheaper.

The 1950s and 1960s can therefore either be seen as the first period in which there was a fruitful coalescence of the organisational and humanitarian perceptions of old age as a social problem, acting to the benefit of both the public purse and of the welfare and happiness of the elderly; or as a period in which contemporary trends in social thought directed against institutionalisation could be exploited by policy makers to mask a continuing concern to reduce the burden of caring for the elderly. Whatever the actual or imputed motivations of policy makers, I would argue that the enthusiastic advocacy of rehabiliation and community care was based to some extent on fallacious premises. I will discuss this point below after sketching in some more recent trends.

Late 1960s to 1976

After a plethora of reports specifically on the care of the aged, overt interest in the aged as a major social problem died down in the late 1960s. This may be attributable to an assumption that the 'community care solution' had solved the organisational and humanitarian problems, and/or to the discovery or rediscovery of other social problems such as child poverty, single parenthood, and over-population.

However, the concept or practice of community care came under increasing criticism from observers and pressure groups. Downie (1972), for example, pointed out that problems such as 'bed-blocking' by chronically ill elderly people, or their 'misplacement' in the wrong sort

Old Age as a Social Problem

of unit, were less of a problem than had been supposed in the early 1960s, and commented on the uncritical acceptance of some of the unsubstantiated assumptions of the community care policy. The lack of provision in the community was criticised in the mass media,[16] and the health authorities started concentrating again on geriatric hospital provision for long-stay as well as rehabilitative care.[17]

In the last year or two there is evidence that attention has again been directed towards the elderly and the social problem they pose from the organisational perspective.[6] With a focus on the economic ills of the country, there has also been a recent revival of the concept of community care, under a new guise — that of self-care as a way of reducing the social costs of the health services.[18]

Discussion

I have tried to show above that, within official conceptions of old age as a social problem, there have been variations in the relative emphasis placed upon organisational and humanitarian concerns. There have not only been changes in whether old age is perceived to be socially problematic, but also in what sort of social problem it is perceived to be. Such varying definitions and perceptions are not only of academic interest: consequences of such definitions when translated into specific policy proposals are interesting and important sociological and social issues.

I have argued that there has been seen to be a tension between the organisational and humanitarian perspectives and the recipes for action deriving from them, the literature of the 1940s containing the most clear statement of this tension. During the 1950s and 1960s the official literature seemed to portray community care as a solution to this tension, rehabilitation and community care being described as being in the interests both of individual old people and of the national economy. I would suggest that this optimism was based on a number of fallacies, and that the tension still remains.

On the organisational level it seems that the beliefs that community care is cheaper than institutional care, and that rehabilitative efforts will reduce social costs in the long run, are dubious. Belief in the first point was based on comparisons between a relatively *high* standard of institutional care and a relatively *low* standard of community care. Careful controlled studies of the costs and benefits of alternative forms of care have not been undertaken (Downie, 1972), though some are now proposed, but there is some evidence that community care at a level recognised as adequate may be just as costly, even if not more so, than institutional care. Furthermore, in these sorts of calculations the *indirect* social costs are often ignored in favour of the easily quantified direct social costs. Discharging elderly people from hospitals may merely transfer the burden of care from one sector to another — from the hospital sector on to families, neighbours and voluntary organisations as well as on to the local authority services. The fact that the burden of care may well be placed on unpaid amateurs instead of paid professionals does not necessarily mean that there are no social costs.

Further, the meaning and components of 'community care' have rarely been defined with any rigour. It is unclear, for example, why living in a half-way house or private hostel should be classified as 'community care' and living in a residential home or hospital be classified as 'institutional' and therefore, by implication, as 'non-community care'. The 'community', qua taxpayer, subsidises all these forms of care, and the fact that the money may come under different budget headings does not alter this fact.

The assumption of short-term investment for a long-run reduction in social costs has never appeared to work for health and welfare services, and there would appear to be good theoretical reasons for such investment *increasing* later social costs. Beveridge appears to have been in error in assuming that initial investment in health services would in the long term reduce costs by lessening the reservoir of disease and incapacity requiring attention. Rather, as Powell (1966) suggests, it seems more plausible to believe that 'Every advance in medical science creates new needs that did not exist until the means of meeting them came into existence, or at least into the realms of the possible' (p. 26); and that 'Improvement in expectation of survival results in lives that demand further medical care' (p. 27). The introduction of rehabilitative techniques 'uncovers' a hitherto unnoticed group of potential recipients of those techniques; as standards rise, so do expectations of what can be achieved, resulting in an increase in demand and expenditure; and even if rehabilitative techniques allow the elderly to be discharged back into the community, we are all mortal and are likely to need further medical care at a later stage and perhaps for longer than we would have done without the initial rehabilitative effort.[19]

On the humanitarian level, the assumption that the old prefer to lead independent lives in their own homes was never examined. Such a preference tended to be imputed to them by younger observers and policy makers, often based on the poor conditions discovered in institutions. While it might be correct that the majority of the elderly would prefer to live independently in their own homes if they were physically fit and financially secure, if these conditions are not met then many might prefer to be looked after in a hospital or home.[20] While not overstressing the significance of the point, it is interesting that the Phillips Report on the one hand stated, as a matter of common knowledge, that old people prefer to live independent lives, and on the other hand stressed the need to *encourage* the elderly to stay in their own homes (para. 264). The question of whether the elderly prefer living at home or in institutions is currently rather academic; not only is there no strong body of evidence as to preferences either way, but conditions are not such that realistic comparisons are possible. If long-term planning were to be based on the expressed desires of old people, one would have to ask hypothetical questions of most of them, such as 'given money, which would you prefer,' or 'given adequate domiciliary facilities and housing, and sufficient places in residential care, what would you choose.'

In conclusion, therefore, it seems that the optimism of the 1950s and 1960s was rather naive, and I would argue that the tension between the two perspectives is a persisting feature of policies towards the aged. I would also suggest that acknowledgement of this tension should be made when examining official policy. Waller (1936) argued that 'The humanitarian often argues for his reforms on the basis of considerations which are consonant with the organisational mores but alien to the spirit of humanitarianism: he advocates a new system of poor relief, saying it will be cheaper, while really he is hoping that it will prove more humane.' (1971 edition, p. 99.) I would suggest that the reverse is also possible: policies designed from an organisational perspective may be presented in humanitarian terms in the hope that this will render them more acceptable. Such a humanitarian rhetoric may mask underlying definitions of the problem and recipes for action which are fundamentally organisational in nature. This and the above points are of relevance not only to old age, but also to other problems of chronicity and incapacity, and the issues here raised may be of increasing importance as such conditions assume greater proportional significance within national morbidity patterns. I would also suggest that these issues are of current significance in the light of recent proposals for future priorities in the health and social services.[18]

Notes

1. For example, Fuller and Myers, 1941; Becker, 1963, 1966; Blumer, 1971;
2. See for example Schur, 1962 and Lindesmith, 1965 on the 'problems' drug addiction may pose for different groups.
3. See: the Report of the Royal Commission of the Aged Poor (1895); the Report of the Committee on Old Age Pensions (1898); Report of the House of Commons Select Committee on the Cottage Homes Bill (1899); the Report of the House of Commons Select Committee on the Aged Deserving Poor (1899); the Majority and Minority Reports of the Royal Commission on the Poor Laws and the Relief of Distress (1909), the Old Age Pensions Act of 1908.
4. As expressed, for example, in: the Beveridge Report (1942); the foundation of the Medical Society for the Care of the Elderly in 1947; Royal Commission on Population (1949); The Phillips Report (1954) and the Boucher Report (1957).
5. For example, Townsend, 1957, 1964; Townsend and Wedderburn, 1965; Shenfield, 1957; Richardson, 1964.
6. This concern has been manifest within the MRC, Department of Health and Social Security, the Scottish Home and Health Department, and the EEC. See also note 18.
7. Similarly, the 1895 Royal Commission noted that: 'The number of aged poor who seek public relief, while still very large, has much lessened in proportion in the last 30 years.' (1895, para. LXXXVII.)
8. See, for example, the activities and reports of Child Poverty Action Group; Family Income Supplement, Finer Report of 1974, 'Gingerbread', Mothers in Action, 'Shelter'.
9. For example, the following scale of relief was instituted at Shifnal:

		per week
Males,	under 60	2s. 0d.
Males,	over 60	2s. 6d.
Males,	over 70	3s. 0d.
Females,	under 60	1s. 6d.
Females,	over 60	2s. 0d.
Females,	over 70	2s. 0d.
Widows		1s. 6d.
Widows with children – for each child		1s. 6d.

(Quoted in Majority Report of the 1909 Royal Commission, para. 334.)

10. 'By associating the respectable and disreputable in institutions without classification, a sense of wrong is aroused in the minds of those with good character.' (1909, Part IX, para. 97.)
11. It can be noted that the Old Age Pension Act of 1908 was non-contributory, i.e. it gave every British National of twenty years residence a pension as of right from exchequer funds on reaching the age of 70, subject to certain exclusions. It thus represented an official commitment to provide pensions out of general taxation, thereby incurring direct social costs.
12. In particular, the Cowley Road Hospital, Oxford; the West Middlesex Hospital; and the Foresthall Hospital, Glasgow. Described in Felstein, 1969.
13. Even before this suggested reduction, residential provision in both homes and hospitals had been reduced. Davis (1971) points out that the rate of

Old Age as a Social Problem

increase in provision required to maintain the same proportion of the elderly by age, sex and marital status in care in either hospitals or residential homes in 1961 as in 1951 was 10½ per cent p.a.: the actual increase was no more than 5.7 per cent p.a.

14. Between 1966 and 1968, when the 'community care' concept was at its peak of popularity, the number of full-time home helps, home nurses, and health visitors declined in England and Wales (Annual Report of Ministry of Health and Social Security, 1969).

15. It found that in 1954-5 the cost of providing domiciliary care per case varied from £2 14s. 0d. to £9 15s. 0d., compared with the average weekly cost of institutional care of £6 12s. 0d. for chronic sick hospitals and £4 9s. 8d. for local authority homes (National Corporation for Old People, Ninth Annual Report, pp. 10-14, quoted in Hall, 1965, p. 293).

16. For a recent example, note the 'Nationwide' television programme on Monday, 16 February 1976, which dealt with mentally ill or subnormal persons discharged from hospital in Birmingham. In the programme the term 'decanting' was used as if it had a taken-for-granted meaning for persons in the field, to describe the 'dumping' of ex-hospital patients on a community with inadequate resources. On the same evening 'Panorama' discussed a similar problem with reference to the mentally ill and retarded in Broadstairs.

17. See, for example, Department of Health and Social Security Annual Report 1971; and the Scottish Home and Health Department's Report for 1974.

18. See, for example, the interview with Dr David Owen reported in *The Times* of 9 February 1976. Dr Owen emphasised the importance of preventive medicine, the use of volunteers in the community, and self-care as a means of reducing the costs of the NHS. He also discussed these themes, and the social costs of the elderly, in his address to the BSA Annual Conference at Manchester, April 1976. See also, of course, the White Paper on the Government's plans for reducing public expenditure, the Consultative Document on Prevention and Health (DHSS) and the proposals for Health and Personal Social Services in England (DHSS).

19. In the BBC television programme 'The Changing Face of Medicine' shown on 20 November 1975, there was a discussion of the elderly in which it was stated that diseases such as rheumatism and arthritis would be curable in the year 2000. The film showed 80 year olds dancing to the 'Pink Floyd', and stressed how the elderly would be able to live active lives into their eighties. It failed to inform us of what such persons would eventually die; assuming them still to be mortal, they would presumably merely develop incapacitating and/or fatal diseases in their nineties instead of seventies and eighties.

20. For those who can afford it, residential care has always been *chosen* by a substantial number of old people even if they do not 'require' it on the grounds of incapacity. There are extensive waiting lists for long-stay hospital beds and for local authority homes and evidence of people wishing admission to such institutions but not even bothering to apply because the scarcity of places is publicly known – this suggests some demand from the elderly.

References

Abel Smith, B. and Townsend, P. (1965), *The Poor and the Poorest* (London, Bell).
Barton, R. (1959), *Institutional Neurosis* (Bristol, John Wright & Sons).
Becker, H. S. (1963), *Outsiders: Studies in the Sociology of Deviance* (New York, Free Press of Glencoe).
Becker, H. S. (ed.) (1966), *Social Problems: A Modern Approach* (New York, John Wiley & Sons).
Bernard, J. (1957), *Social Problems at Mid Century: Role, Status and Stress in a Context of Abundance* (New York, Dryden Press).
Blumer, H. (1971), 'Social Problems as Collective Behaviour', *Social Problems* 18 (3), pp. 298-306.
Bowlby, J. (1951), *Maternal Care and Mental Health* (Geneva, WHO).
Bull, D. and Townsend, P. (1971), *Family Poverty: Programme for the Seventies* (London, Gerald Duckworth & Co.).
Davis, B. P., Barton, A. J., McMillan, I. S. and Williamson, U. K. (1971), *Variations in Services for the Aged: A Causal Analysis*, Occasional Papers on Social Administration No. 40 (London, Bell & Sons).
Downie, B. D. (1972), 'The Elderly in Scottish Hospitals 1961-66', Scottish Home and Health Department, *Scottish Health Service Studies No. 21* (Edinburgh, HMSO).
Felstein, I. (1969), *Later Life: Geriatrics Today and Tomorrow* (London, Routledge & Kegan Paul).
Fuller, R. C. and Myers, R. R. (1941), 'The Natural History of a Social Problem', *A.S.R.*, June, pp. 321-8.
Government Publications

1834	*Report of the Royal Commission on the Administration and Practical Operation of the Poor Laws.*
1873-4	*Report on the Administration of Outdoor Relief in the Metropolis*, in Third Annual Report of the Local Government Board, 1873-4.
1895	*Report of the Royal Commission on the Aged Poor*, Cmnd. 7684 (London, HMSO).
1898	*Report of the Committee on Old Age Pensions*, Cmnd. 8911 (London, HMSO).
1899	*Report of the House of Commons Select Committee on The Cottage Homes Bill* (House of Commons, No. 271 of 1899).
1899	*Report of the House of Commons Select Committee on Aged Deserving Poor* (House of Commons, No. 296 of 1899).
1909	*Report of the Royal Commission on the Poor Laws and Relief of Distress*, Cmnd. 4499 (London, printed for His Majesty's Stationery Office by Wyman and Sons Ltd.).
1942	Beveridge, Sir W., *Social Insurance and Allied Services*, Cmnd. 6404 (London, HMSO).
1949	*Royal Commission on Population*, Cmnd. 7695 (London, HMSO).
1954	Ministry of Pensions and National Insurance, *National Insurance Retirement Pensions, Reasons given for Retiring or Continuing at Work* (London, HMSO).
1954	Phillips Report, *Report of the Committee on the Economic and Financial Problems of the Provision for Old Age*, Cmnd. 9333 (London, HMSO).
1956	Guillebaud Report, *Report of the Committee of Enquiry into the Cost of the National Health Service*, Cmnd. 9663 (London, HMSO).
1957	Boucher Report, *Report on Services Available for the Chronic Sick*

            and Elderly, Reports on Public Health and Medical Subjects, No. 98 (London, HMSO).
1962   Hospital Plan for England and Wales Cmnd. 1604 (London, HMSO).
1963   Ministry of Health, Health and Welfare: the Development of Community Care, Cmnd. 1973 (London, HMSO).
1969   Ministry of Health and Social Security, Annual Report 1968, Cmnd. 4100 (London, HMSO).
1972   Department of Health and Social Security, Annual Report 1971, Cmnd, 5019 (London, HMSO).
1974   Finer Report, Report of the Committee on One Parent Families, Cmnd. 5629 (London, HMSO).
1975   Scottish Home and Health Department, Health Services in Scotland: Report for 1974, Cmnd. 6052 (Edinburgh, HMSO).
1976   Department of Health and Social Security, 'Prevention and Health: Everybody's Business'. A Consultative Document prepared jointly by the Health Departments of Great Britain and Northern Ireland.
1976   Department of Health and Social Security, 'Priorities for Health and Personal Social Services in England'.

Hall, M. P. (1965), The Social Services of Modern England (London, Routledge & Kegan Paul).

Harrington, M. (1963), The Other America: Poverty in the United States (Harmondsworth, Middx, Penguin).

Lemert, E. M. (1951), Social Pathology (New York, McGraw-Hill).

Lindesmith, A. R. (1965), The Addict and the Law (Bloomington, Indiana University Press).

Parker, J. (1962), Local Health and Welfare Services (London, Allen & Unwin).

Powell, J. E. (1966), A New Look at Medicine and Politics (London, Pitman Medical).

Richardson, I. M. (1964), Age and Need: A Study of Older People in North East Scotland (Edinburgh, E. & S. Livingstone).

Schur, E. M. (1962), Narcotic Addiction in Britain and America: The Impact of Public Policy (Bloomington, Indiana University Press).

Shenfield, B. E. (1957), Social Policies for Old Age: A Review of Social Provision for Old Age in Great Britain (London. Routledge & Kegan Paul).

Townsend, P. (1957), The Family Life of Old People (London, Routledge & Kegan Paul).

Townsend, P. (1964), The Last Refuge: A Survey of Residential Institutions and Homes for the Aged in England and Wales (London, Routledge & Kegan Paul).

Waller, W. (1936), 'Social Problems and the Mores', A.S.R., December, pp. 924-30.

Medical sociology has still to fulfil its potential in many areas. None is more neglected, yet offers us greater understanding of the present day, than historical studies of medical knowledge. We are fortunate that the papers in this volume do not always represent the typical, but, as with the following paper, are the product of successful research in new directions. The two preceeding papers offered an analysis of the development of ideas drawn from more than a century of medical thought, tracing changes through a series of reformers and reformist ideals. This paper takes a similar perspective but, by comparison, covers a briefer time span. Here, the author presents us with a detailed analysis of one man, one innovation and its influence.

Taking as his example the field of psychiatry, Fears argues that much can be gained by identifying the normative origins and logical nature of current psychiatric ideals of moral prescription and social control. He identifies the introduction of 'moral treatment' in the early 1800s as a key influence in the shift in psychiatric ideology, and carefully locates the ideas to both the time and the person. The strength of Fears' work lies in the successful manner in which he tackles the question of why moral treatment emerged at one particular time in history. While attributing its introduction to one man, Samuel Tukes, Fears nevertheless eschews the 'great man' theory of historical explanation. Instead, the various arguments for its emergence and acceptance at that time are dealt with in turn. Ideas for innovation, it is suggested, are never created in a void but spring from a variety of sources, from neglected ideas or out of vogue theories. Tukes, we find, placed high premium on his own Quaker values which moulded his world, and in turn, affected the praxis of the asylum for the mentally ill which Tukes ran.

By using the sociology of knowledge to explore some of the origins of current psychiatric thought Fears offers us an historical picture of medical innovation. At the same time, he highlights the contemporary importance of such an account. The influence of Tukes' ideas of moral treatment can be seen in present-day psychiatric rhetoric and practice.

M.R.

THERAPEUTIC OPTIMISM AND THE TREATMENT OF THE INSANE:
Some Comments on the Interpretation of Psychiatric Reform at the End of the Eighteenth Century

Michael Fears

Psychiatry has been subjected to a number of criticisms in the last decade or so, often on the grounds that as social practice it is not objective and value free, as it often purports to be, but contains within itself a large amount of evaluational and moral content. In other words to treat someone as insane or mentally ill involves not only the use of scientific knowledge but also the invocation of social and moral norms of how people ought to act. Given the increasing influence of psychiatric knowledge it is surprising that so few attempts have been made to uncover just what those norms are and how it is that psychiatry has been able to reify them into apparently objective knowledge. Thomas Szasz's *Manufacture of Madness*,[1] Ronald Laing's *Politics of Experience*,[2] and Michel Foucault's *Madness and Civilization*[3] are three works which have become widely known for the provocative way they have stimulated debate of these issues. All three have been severely criticised on a number of grounds, not least that they are short on evidence. Nevertheless they have raised questions about the nature of psychiatric knowledge which at the very least have disturbed the complacency of orthodox psychiatry. At the same time it must be said that these critiques have often been less than influential because the force of their criticism appeared to rest on an assumption that a psychiatry could exist that did not involve social control and moral prescription. The utopianism of the 1960s is now over, but that is no reason why the radical critiques which that period stimulated, should not themselves be placed on a more stable basis.

The following paper, while accepting many of the criticisms that have been made (and especially those by Foucault), attempts to replace what it sees as the idealist perspective in that work by one grounded in the sociology of knowledge. In other words 'We set out from real active men, and on the basis of their real life-process we demonstrate the development of the ideological reflexes and echoes of this life-process.'[4]

This approach, while lacking the rhetorical splendour of Foucault's work, should provide an addition to our knowledge of 'what happened' for one particular period in the history of psychiatry. Only in this way can we understand the precise mechanisms by which 'the social construction of reality' takes place.[5] The 'real active men' that this paper concerns itself with are the reformers at the beginning of the nineteenth century who were responsible for introducing and developing the therapeutic programme known as 'Moral Treatment'.[6]

'Moral Treatment' was unheard of before 1800. By 1850 its use was proclaimed in every institution for the insane and every textbook or treatise on insanity had a chapter on it. Before 1800 provision of care for the insane was predominantly on a small and *ad hoc* basis, locally planned and relying on individual initiative. The chances of a mentally ill person obtaining specialist attention depended primarily on how much money he had or on how dangerous he was believed to be. After 1850 statutory provision was made for everyone certified as insane, usually in large public asylums which were centrally administered and publicly financed. Moral treatment is perhaps not the most important feature of that half-century but without its influence the changes would have been made in a markedly different direction.

The first English writer to use the words 'Moral Treatment' in reference to his own practice was Samuel Tuke, who in 1813 listed the first principle of moral treatment as 'By what means the power of the patient to control the disorder, is strengthened and assisted'.[7] Samuel Tuke was not a doctor but the treasurer to a small private asylum near York which was opened by his grandfather, William Tuke (who also had no medical training) in 1796. This asylum, known as 'The Retreat' was originally opened solely for members of the Society of Friends who had become insane. All the Tuke family were themselves devout Quakers. What made the Retreat famous was the publication in 1813 of a book written by Samuel Tuke and called, simply, *Description of the Retreat*. Almost unanimously, support was given by all who concerned themselves with *improving* the condition of the insane, to implementing the Tukes' ideas on moral treatment.

It is in the seventeen years between 1796 and the publication of the *Description* in 1813 that moral treatment was developed at the Retreat. The *Description* does not give an account of that development; indeed it views moral treatment as an accomplished fact; but it is possible by looking at the early reports and visitors' accounts of the early years to gain a fairly clear picture of the changing practice.[8]

The first years of the Retreat's existence do not appear to have been easy ones. Because of the attractiveness of a specifically Quaker institution for the insane, Friends from all over the country immediately started to transfer their relatives from other madhouses. The effect of this can be seen in a comment made by William Tuke in 1798 that 'out of 23 cases in the House, all of them, except two or three, were, at their admission, of so long standing as to be considered incurable'.[9] One patient committed suicide, others ran away. Some of the servants proved inadequate for the job and had to be dismissed. Less than two months after the Retreat opened the Superintendent died. Tuke took on the job himself on a temporary basis and it was over a year later before a replacement was found in George Jepson, ex-weaver, unqualified lay doctor, and above all, a devout Quaker. He remained until his death twenty-six years later.

The Retreat employed a consultant physician to advise on appropriate therapies, and in the early years the conventional wisdom was, albeit cautiously, applied. Bleedings, purges and vomits, the unholy trinity of eighteenth-century therapeutics, were tried at the Retreat and fairly quickly discarded. Whereas a qualified mad-doctor would be likely, because of his theoretical understanding of pathology, to continue in using bleedings even if any particular case was unsuccessful, for the Tukes it was the success or failure of a therapy in any particular case that led them to modify their therapeutic programme.

This principle can be seen at work in their use of fear. It was a popular idea throughout the eighteenth century that the mental patient could be frightened into submission. John Brown, lecturer in medicine at Edinburgh University, wrote in 1788 that '. . . the patient should be struck with fear and terror, and driven, in his state of insanity, to despair'. For Brown, mania was 'sthenic apyrexia' or non-inflammatory excitement. Its cure consisted not in tranquillity but in exhausting 'the high commotion of spirits'. Therefore, maintained Brown, 'As a remedy against the great excitement of the organs of voluntary motion, the labour of draft-cattle should be imposed on him, and assiduously continued, his diet should be the poorest possible, and his drink only water'.[10] This was heroic medicine at its worst and yet at first glance there is much in common between this and a report we have of the methods used at the Retreat when it was first opened. 'Fear', we are told, was 'the great principle by which the insane [were] to be governed . . . [and] in some cases of violent excitement, the cudgel and the whip were the most suitable instruments of coercion.'[11]

But, as with the more physical remedies, each use of fear at the Retreat was assessed on its individual merits. A Swiss doctor who visited the Retreat in 1798 described the therapeutic programme there in the following way:

> You will perceive that in the moral treatment of the insane, they do not consider them as absolutely deprived of reason; or, in other words, as inaccessible to the motives of fear, hope, feeling, and honour. It appears, that they consider them rather as children, who have too much strength, and who make a dangerous use of it. Their punishments and rewards must be immediate, since that which is distant has no effect upon them . . . Subject them at first; encourage them afterwards, employ them, and render their employment agreeable by attractive means.[12]

This sort of 'positive management' had been experimented with before, notably at Manchester Lunatic Asylum. The physician there wrote in the same decade how 'the management of hope and apprehension in the patients, forms the most useful part of discipline. Small favours, the show of confidence, and apparent distinction, accelerate recovery.' One way the physician at Manchester thought this might be achieved was through segregating the good patients from the bad. 'It has long been my wish,' he wrote, 'that a room might be appropriated in our hospital, to convalescents; and that the priviledge of admission to it might be made the reward of regular behaviour among the patients. Such a distinction would act powerfully in creating a habit of self-restraint, the first salutary operation in the mind of a lunatic.'[13]

What the Tukes did was to integrate the logic of this reasoning into the therapeutic milieu they were trying to establish at the Retreat. Thus it can be seen in their use of fear, and also in the way they developed the use of physical restraints such as the straitjacket. At that time the strait-jacket (or strait waistcoat as it was called) was a fairly new invention, but the principle was old enough — to restrain the madman when he was violent so as to prevent him from hurting himself and others. The use made of it at the Retreat, while not unique, does show the subtle way in which the Tukes were developing old methods for new aims. The following comments were made of one unruly patient: '. . . he strikes the other patients if not well watched and has often attempted to strike his physician. On such occasions it is found proper to put on the strait waistcoat for a day or two to make him ashamed of his conduct.'[14] The strait-jacket has become here a punishment, a subtle means by which the patient is encouraged to reflect on his condition and, most importantly, to attempt to control himself.

Fear was one means of controlling the patients' insane behaviour but it was very crude and, as the Tukes realised, cruel to the patients who were far more sensitive to pain than they were usually given credit for. Far more effective than the use of fear was the manipulation of something the Tukes called the patient's 'desire for esteem'. 'When properly cultivated,' Tuke wrote in the *Description*, 'it leads many to struggle to conceal and overcome their morbid propensities; and, at least, materially assists them in confining their deviations, within such bounds, as do not make them obnoxious to the family.'[15] Means by which this desire for esteem were cultivated included tea parties. 'All who attend,' wrote Tuke, 'dress in their best clothes, and vie with each other in politeness and propriety.'[16] Patients of the 'higher class' who behaved well enough were allowed to eat their meals with the superintendent as a reward for good conduct.

The most important aspect of this therapeutic family was given to the value of work. In Tuke's words again, 'Of all the modes by which the patients may be induced to restrain themselves, regular employment is perhaps the most generally efficacious.'[17] The type of work that the patients were encouraged to engage in depended on what they had been doing outside. The Retreat was not just for rich Quakers. It was opened for lunatics from all classes of society. But of course the divisions in 'normal' society were reflected in the institution that was designed to return its patients to it. Segregation was enforced, both by sex and 'rank' in society, as well as by degree of illness. The few upper-class patients, for instance, could live with their own servants and were not expected to engage in productive labour. For them, 'regular employment' meant regular exercise of the body through walks in the garden and exercise of the mind through the useful study of 'mathematics and natural science'. The 'lower class' patients were expected to help in manual labour in the garden, helping the attendants with refractory patients, and in domestic chores. A hint of the extent to which this employment was enforced can be seen in the comments of one patient's relative: '. . . if he [the patient] was under strict discipline' this correspondent wrote, 'I am fully of the mind he be made to earn his bread.'[18]

With the publication of the *Description* in 1813, its microscopic example of a complete model society was taken up and applied to other asylums, both public and private. For example, Samuel Tuke himself was called upon to give advice in the planning of the pauper asylum for the West Riding of Yorkshire at Wakefield. He recommended the installation of looms so that the patients could continue with the same 'regular employment' they did outside. The suggestion was taken up so enthusiastically that, two years after the asylum's opening, all the clothes and shoes for the patients were made by themselves. Many influential people visited the Retreat and praised this new experiment in the care of the insane. Sydney Smith reviewed Samuel Tuke's *Description* for the *Edinburgh Review* and wrote 'We have little doubt that this is the best managed asylum for the insane that has ever yet been established.'[19] Other examples could be given but are not really necessary; the influence of what happened at the Retreat is undisputed. The question that needs to be answered is why this was so.

One frequently given answer is that the regime at the Retreat was based on humanitarian principles. Certainly if we compare it with some of the alternative provisions for the insane its mildness is obvious. For instance, the other main provision in York was the York Lunatic Asylum, a hospital founded by public subscription in 1777, but by 1814 apparently little more than a device for making its physician a rich man. Extreme overcrowding, neglect of physical ailments, the rape of female patients, beatings, as well as the constant physical restraint and lack of any medical or moral treatment — such are the images against which the experiment at the Retreat is constantly and to some extent justifiably juxtaposed.

But why, if kindness was the only aim, was such an intense effort made to resocialise the patients into a particular version of normality? The Retreat never instituted kindness for kindness' sake — it was always for a purpose. Nowhere in the Tukes' writings do we hear of straightforward compassion for the sick; gentle methods yes, but always to achieve something. The medical superintendent expressed it quite unambiguously in 1841: 'The primary object . . . has been that of cultivating in the patient the moral sense of right and wrong, the power of self restraint and the remaining mental faculties as much as practicable.'[20]

A further answer that is sometimes given as to why moral treatment emerged when it did is that the management of the insane has always been a problem for those who concern themselves with their care, but that because a particular view of the nature of insanity was held up to the end of the eighteenth century, it was not possible for management to be reformed before then. This argument draws on the image we have of the eighteenth century as the age of reason, with the madman as the man without rational thought and so necessarily less than human. The madman was to be shocked back to normality by cold baths, or his fever reduced by bleeding; there was no point in appealing to his sense of understanding because it was that which had been destroyed by his madness. This model of insanity is usually held to be backed up by the contemporary idea that mental disorder was a symptom of brain disease. Almost without exception the medical theories in the eighteenth century stressed that insanity was a physical disease of the brain. Non-physical causes were accepted but once physical degeneration had set in, what was the point of using non-physical methods in curing it? The case is clearly put by a physician to a county asylum:

> From morbid anatomy we learn that in ninety-five cases out of a hundred of the deranged patients examined after death, the structure of the brain is materially injured by chronic inflammation of its investing membranes or by an effusion of water into its ventricles. It must be evident to every individual possessing common sense, that water in the ventricles and chronic inflammation of its membranes, can neither be obviated nor cured by moral treatment.[21]

So physicians, accepting the Cartesian separation of mind and body saw no point in appealing to one to affect the other.

Against this background the Tukes are presumed to be naive empiricists, holding no commitment to a particular theory of disease, and thus being able to try out methods of therapy which accepted a universal humanity. In the words of Kathleen Jones' *History of the Mental Health Services*, the Retreat 'evolved a form of treatment based, not on the scanty medical knowledge of the time, but on Christianity and common-sense'.[22] According to this version of events it was rather fortuitous that soon after moral treatment became publicised the science of phrenology appeared. As Bynum puts it in a recent account of this period:

> The phrenological concept of mental functions circumvented the traditional Cartesian framework and permitted phrenologists to

refer simultaneously to the experienced mental state and its underlying physiological counterpart. The effectiveness of moral therapy could be understood both in terms of psychological benefit and the concomitant hypertrophy of the stimulated areas of the cerebral cortex.[23]

Doctors were thus encouraged to attempt the amelioration of any disordered mental state either by direct moral treatment of the disordered faculty, or if it was believed to be too diseased, by building up the faculties that were not damaged.

This is one account of what happened, which relies for its explanatory power on the role of specialised knowledge. But it is not adequate as an explanation, if only because it is so selective of the medical theories of the time. There *were* medical theories around which allowed for a sophisticated management of the insane, and one of them, the doctrine of the passions, was precisely the theory which Pinel, the originator of the term 'moral treatment', used to justify his practice in France.[24]

Pinel's argument was that since madness was caused by the passions getting out of hand, what better way was there of regaining sanity, than by trying to control or manipulate those same passions? The word 'passions' is not meant at all metaphorically. In Pinel's usage it refers to the moral affections which medical theory for centuries had accepted were part of man's endowments. What Pinel did which was so different was to use the same theory optimistically — to say that even if there was some permanent damage which could not be cured, the insane person did not have to be written off as useless.

Samuel Tuke also used the word 'passions' in his work but without attempting to support any particular medical theory. He did read a number of treatises on insanity before writing the *Description* and he did with them what any other specialist in insanity had done. He chose from among them whatever would serve his interests. For instance, a physician who wanted to could keep on referring back to the Greek authorities, or to the most traditional practices to justify his actions.

The philosophy expressed not only at the Retreat but in Manchester Lunatic Hospital and at a few private madhouses was an overriding and pragmatic commitment to trying anything if it seemed to work. Bleedings were tried but discarded if found to be ineffective. Seen in this light the knowledge of phrenology provided an intellectual justification for therapeutic optimism, but the impetus for cautious experimentation in the treatment of the insane had been around much longer. Part of a sociological explanation of the treatment of insanity at this time must lie in the changing structure of the medical profession, in the different professional characteristics of men like Thomas Monro, physician of Bethlem, or Ferriar, the physician at Manchester Lunatic Hospital. Their whole approach to what the 'practice of medicine' meant was different, and can be traced to a number of external causes.[25] My primary concern here, though, is moral treatment and its meaning within the Retreat.

Part of this meaning can be found in the religious beliefs of the Quakers. Like other eighteenth-century groups they held that the spirit of God existed in every man – the basis of human nature was this universal quality. But this Spirit could only be recognised, or to put it another way, each man's moral character could only be realised, if his animal passions were kept under control. So although the Spirit of God was held to exist in every man, it was every man's duty to make sure it had the opportunity of being expressed. One contemporary commentator on the Quakers has left us a vivid picture of what happened when the passions got out of hand in card playing:

> I have been told [he wrote] that large drops of sweat have fallen from their faces though they were under no bodily exertions. Now what must have been the state of their minds when the card in question proved decisive of their loss? Reason must unquestionably have fled; and it must have been succeeded instantly either by fury or despair . . . It is not necessary to have recourse to the theory of the human mind to anticipate the consequences that would be likely to result from such an extreme excitement of the passions.[26]

Again we are back with the passions, this time in a religious context, and again they are taking us close to madness. In the Retreat everything was excised that might cause such immoderate expressions of man's baser nature, and everything was encouraged that would help the patients to express their true moral character.

There is no reason to disagree with the Tukes' religious commitments but there is every reason not to be content with this as a total explanation. The Quakers' moral world, to put it bluntly, did not exist in a vacuum, but in a society in a state of fundamental change; What they counted as morally good, or bad, must be related to that change.

One possibility is to see within the Retreat the resemblance of a return to nature. In the *Description* are frequent references to such factors as pollution-free air, the view over unspoilt country, the fertile garden, and the therapeutic value of working on the land. Michel Foucault has emphasised this quality in his comments on the Tukes: 'All the imaginary strength of the simple life, of rustic happiness, of a return to the seasons are summoned here together in order to preside at the recovery of sanity. Madness, in conformity with eighteenth century ideas, is seen as a sickness not of nature, nor of man himself, but of society.'[27]

There is ample confirmation of this in the writings of many people in this period. Across the whole range of political attitudes we can see the emergence of arcadian imagery as the new demands of industrialisation are confronted. The social problems that seemed to be endemic in the new towns presented a stark antithesis to the apparent social and moral order of the old rural communities. But while this was a common theme of the time, the Tukes do not overemphasise it. Given the fact that York was not an industrial town, the Tukes' commitment to a rural way of life cannot have quite the significance that Foucault gives it. The *Description* does not plead for a return to a 'natural' moral order, it merely states its existence within a world where that moral order had not yet been destroyed.

One normative order that is pleaded for more strongly is that of the family. From contemporary accounts, William Tuke appears as a stern patriarchal figure, presiding over the dinner table in his joint authority as superintendent and as father. Because of the Retreat's small size (36 patients in 1800, 49 in 1812) a close familial environment would not have been difficult to maintain. In the *Description* Samuel Tuke compared the insane to children, especially in the similarity of the 'judicious treatment'[28] they both needed. And on the use of fear he stressed that '... it is not allowed to be excited, beyond that degree which naturally arises from the necessary regulations of the family'.[29]

What were the values expressed in this family in which instead of children it was the insane who were to learn the proper way to live? According to Foucault the aim was:

> A strict family, without any weaknesses or complacency, but just, conforming to the fine image of the biblical family ... In the Retreat the human group is escorted back to the most original and pure of all forms ... where society and nature both came into view together and where it achieves an immediate truth that all the history of man has only confused.[30]

My own reading of the *Description* allows no such imputation; true, the Quaker moral order saw itself as committed to a timeless and universal truth, but so do all moralities. What makes the Quaker morality so interesting at this time is the way it provides an expression of the precise opposite of timelessness; that is, the current social requirements of its practitioners as active members of their society.

The ideas of right and wrong that the Tukes expressed in the behaviour that they required their patients to emulate were not abstract concepts – they were directly related to the right and wrong behaviour by which the Tukes ordered their own lives. Their idea of mental health was an expression of what they saw as making their own lives materially successful. In other words moral treatment was an embodiment of praxis, of the implicit recognition by the Tukes that the world they lived in was created by themselves, and there was no reason for anyone such as the insane to be excluded from that world. The two major cornerstones of moral treatment were self-discipline and work. It was these that the Tukes saw as cornerstones of their own personal success and which they believed could be successful in the rehabilitation of their patients back to being active, conscious and creative members of society.

William Tuke is not an isolated figure. He stands as a fairly typical member of his class, the traders and small-scale manufacturers who made up the growing urban bourgeoisie. Perhaps Tuke was stricter in his personal life than most but his general aims were those of his contemporaries: through hard work and self-discipline they believed they would be able to achieve the position in society that was closed to them because of their lack of inherited property or title. Before branching out into the treatment of the insane, William Tuke had spent many years as a cocoa merchant and manufacturer, and tea wholesaler. His career was one of gradual success, hampered by the restrictive practices of the East India Tea Company and the York Society of Merchant Adventurers. Against the traditionally sanctioned privileges of these monopolistic bodies, Tuke embodied the aims of free enterprise; the commercial entrepreneur made good.[31]

Besides the general reasons why someone with strong commercial and manufacturing interests should bother to develop moral treatment, there are a number of local reasons, connected with the position of the Quakers in York at that time. The Retreat was opened during the Napoleonic Wars when the Quakers, who refused to fight for pacifist reasons, were accused of being unpatriotic. The conflict this created in their minds led to the idea that 'we can serve our country in no way more availingly', as one Quaker put it, 'than by contributing all that in us lies, to increase the number of meek, humble, and self-denying Christians'.[32] William Tuke was an active and conscientious Quaker, having already founded a school whose aim was to instil the right values in impressionable children. When a Quaker patient died in suspicious circumstances at the York public lunatic asylum it provided just that impetus for Tuke to extend his social construction of reality into the treatment of the insane.

But in the same moment that the Tukes acknowledged their praxis by trying to reproduce it in the asylum they denied it by attempting to reify their example into a universal law of human nature. At times their therapeutic optimism comes close to the work of Robert Owen, who was a far more radical thinker because he explicitly acknowledged the human authorship of his world and attempted to rebuild society on that basis. The Tukes never went that far. In practice they did the same thing; that is, they set up model communities for moral and social education. But whereas Owen admitted his communities were to serve the interests of people aware of their needs the Tukes simultaneously denied the human authorship of their world and looked for universal laws of human nature in religion and science. 'It appears,' said Samuel Tuke, 'to be a providential ordination that our healthy and most agreeable feelings are connected with the employment of our time in the moderately active pursuit of some apparently useful object.'[33] He hedges his bets by continuing to say that even if man's nature was not so constituted, the patients in the asylum come from a background where useful labour is the norm. This repeated appeal to universal explanations is more than a hurried rationalisation. By appealing to 'providential ordination', or to a social norm, or as the phrenologists did, to science, the moral therapists were able to express as a universal value something which was of very recent origin. The ideas that work and self-discipline were major constituents of mental health did not appear before the last part of the eighteenth century. Neither of course did the factory system of production or industrial towns.

The emphasis that the Tukes placed on the value of work also raises an interesting point about their supposed empiricism. They rejected the medical therapies of the time, irrespective of the theoretical respectability they might have, because of their poor practical value in curing insanity. Each therapy was rationally tried on its merits and only discarded after a fair trial. No such methodical concern can be seen in their application of employment as a therapy. Irrespective of the clinical symptoms every patient was directed to carry on with the work they had done before becoming sick — that it would help them was assumed, not demonstrated. This therapy by fiat did not go unnoticed amongst those who had been implicitly criticised by the popular success of the Retreat. John Haslam, apothecary to Bethlem Hospital, commented on the new fashion:

> The different forms of the disease would necessarily require different modes of occupation ... Some skills, and much caution, are also required, to seize the proper time when employment will become beneficial: as I have known many persons relapse, in consequence of having been prematurely, and injudiciously urged to active occupation.[34]

But Haslam was a voice in the wind. English society and the treatment of the insane were both in a process of fundamental change. The Tukes should be seen as one piece in the jigsaw of this change. They used moral treatment in an attempt to consolidate what they saw as worthwhile by producing a mental health which fitted in with the progress of their own lives. This rather narrow conception of mental hygiene, with its dependence on Quaker philosophy, was taken up and developed by other reformers with different interests. But it was precisely because the Tukes denied the social role of the values involved that the ground was laid for two major aspects of Victorian psychiatry. One of these was the degeneration of moral treatment into the euphemism for social control that it became in the enormous Victorian 'bins' where any pretence of praxis was soon abandoned. Although moral treatment was based on an individualist and competitive philosophy there was nothing intrinsic in it to equate it only with the philistine views of the Quakers or the obsession with productive labour that some moral therapists gave it. There were other enthusiasts who used moral treatment to encourage their patients in a wide range of imaginative and creative activities.[35] But its apparent success in creating willing workers made it seem just what many factory owners wanted. As one wrote, 'It is ... excessively the interest of every mill-owner to organize his moral machinery on equally sound principles with his mechanical, for otherwise he will never command the steady hands, watchful eyes, and prompt co-operation, essential to excellence of product.'[36] The Tukes were creating, in the experimental conditions of the Retreat, a prototype of just that moral machinery.

The other aspect of Victorian psychiatry which had its foundations laid at the Retreat was the production of the body of knowledge known as psychiatric theory. The basic claim of this psychiatry to be objective and value free contains within it the ambiguity, initiated by moral treatment, to be both morally neutral and morally better than what went before.

Describing moral treatment in this way is not intended to devalue the attempts at reform by people like the Tukes. The sociology of knowledge, as understood in this paper, is a means by which we can return to our rational control the knowledge that up till now has only existed for us in its reified form, as myth. If human interests lie behind all attempts at reform this is only to say that the world is socially constructed and is infinitely malleable. The Tukes attempted to improve society by extending their values to a group who were previously ignored. But instead of allowing their improvement to be itself transcended, they attempted, like the bourgeois political economists, to ossify the world in their own image. They succeeded very well, but in denying the human authorship of their schemes they forfeited the one possibility of achieving their primary aim – that of tying the treatment of the insane to universal values.

Notes

1. London, Paladin, 1973.
2. Harmondsworth, Penguin, 1967.
3. London, Tavistock, 1967.
4. K. Marx, F. Engels, *The German Ideology* (London, Lawrence and Wishart, 1970), p. 47. Such a claim is of course the promise of a particular methodology, and not the assertion that the work has been done.
5. The phrase is from P. L. Berger and T. Luckmann, *The Social Construction of Reality* (Harmondsworth, Penguin, 1971). The discussion on p. 130 of that work is specifically relevant to the theme of this paper.
6. Because the term 'Moral Treatment' is unfamiliar the phrase has frequently been translated into present-day language. For instance E. T. Carlson and N. Dain write of 'The Psychotherapy that was moral treatment', *Amer. J. Psychiat.*, 117 (1960), pp. 519-24, and W. F. Bynum in 'Rationales for therapy in British Psychiatry 1780-1835', *Med. Hist.*, 18 (1974), pp. 317-34 accepts Carlson and Dain's equation of moral treatment with 'therapeutic efforts which affected the patient's psychology'. There are a number of less 'Whiggish' accounts now beginning to appear, notably Vieda Skultan's introduction to her *Madness and Morals* (London, Routledge & Kegan Paul, 1975) and Andrew Scull's 'From madness to mental illness: medical men as moral entrepreneurs', *Arch. europ. sociol.*

XVI (1975), pp. 218-61. Although these works are not mentioned here again this paper may be seen as engaging in a debate with the issues raised by these writers.
7. S. Tuke, *Description of the Retreat*. Facsimile reprint of 1813 edition with introduction by Richard Hunter and Ida Macalpine (London, Dawsons, 1964), p. 138. (Hereafter referred to as *Descrption*.)
8. I would like to acknowledge the help of Dr D. Smith, Director of the Borthwick Inst., York, in making the archives of the Retreat available to me.
9. *Report of the State of the Institution*, 31 March 1798, p. 9.
10. J. Brown, *The Elements of Medicine* (London, J. Johnson, 1788), Vol. I, p. 52 and Vol. II, p. 168.
11. This is from the anonymous *A Sketch of the Origin, Progress and Present State of the Retreat* (1828), and attributed to Samuel Tuke. It is quoted in A. Walk, 'Some Aspects of the "Moral Treatment" of the insane up to 1854', *J. Mental Science*, 100 (1954), pp. 817-18.
12. Charles de la Rive, quoted, approvingly, in *Description*, p. 223.
13. J. Ferriar, *Medical Histories and Reflections* (Warrington, T. Cadell, 1792-98), Vol. II, pp. 111-12.
14. [W. Tuke] Case notes on John Baker, 24 November 1798.
15. *Description*, p. 157.
16. Ibid., p. 178.
17. Ibid., p. 156.
18. George Withy, letter to W. Tuke, 9 January 1797.
19. *Edinburgh Review* XXIII (April 1814), p. 197.
20. John Thurnam in a *Statistical Report of the Retreat*, quoted in Walk, p. 818.
21. Caleb Crowther, *Some Observations respecting the Management of the Pauper Lunatic Asylum at Wakefield* (Wakefield, Wakefield Journal, 1830), pp. 16-17.
22. Kathleen Jones, *A History of the Mental Health Services* (London, Routledge & Kegan Paul, 1972), p. 45.
23. Bynum, p. 331.
24. For Pinel, see his *Treatise on Insanity* (New York, Hafner Pub. Co., 1962, facsimile copy of 1806 edn.), and K. M. Grange 'Pinel and eighteenth century psychiatry', *Bull. Hist. Med.*, 35 (1961), pp. 442-53.
25. On this cf. N. D. Jewson, 'Medical Knowledge and the Patronage System in 18th century England', *Sociology*, 8 (1974), pp. 369-85, and Scull.
26. T. Clarkson, *A Portraiture of Quakerism* (London, Longmans, 1807), Vol. I, p. 29.
27. This passage does not appear in *Madness and Civilization*, the abridged English translation of *Histoire de la folie a l'age classique*. It is from the second French edition (Paris, Gallimard, 1972), p. 492 (my translation).
28. *Description*, p. 150.
29. Ibid., p. 141.
30. Foucault, pp. 494-5 (my translation).
31. On Tuke's career see W. K. and E. M. Sessions, *The Tukes of York* (London, Friends Home Service Committee, 1971); H. C. Hunt, 'The Life of William Tuke', *J. Friends Hist. Soc.*, XXXIV (1937), pp. 3-18.
32. John Merryweather, 'Epistle to the yearly meeting for 1804', in *Epistles from the yearly meeting of Friends* (London, W. & S. Graves, 1818), p. 516.
33. S. Tuke, introduction to M. Jacobi, *On the Construction and Management of Hospitals for the Insane* (London, J. Churchill, 1841), p. xxix. Compare

this with Robert Owen's 'Human nature its capacities and powers, is yet to be learned by the world. Its faculties are unknown, unappreciated, and therefore misdirected...' (R. Owen, *Life* (New York, A. M. Kelly, 1967, facsimile reprint of 1857 edn., Vol. I, p. 140)).

34. J. Haslam, *Considerations on the Moral Management of Insane Persons* (London, R. Hunter, 1817), p. 72.
35. The most notable is W. A. F. Browne, Medical Superintendent at Crichton Royal, Dumfries. See his *What Asylums Were, Are and Ought to Be* (Edinburgh, A. & C. Black, 1837).
36. Andrew Ure, *The Philosophy of Manufactures* (London, Charles Knight, 1835), p. 417.

In a volume devoted to the development and implementation of medical knowledge, the logical question which must follow papers dealing with the emergence of medical ideas is: how is medical knowledge perpetuated? Some medical information may become available to the lay public, revealed through critical accounts in the mass media or health education. Students entering medical school already have access to this kind of medical disclosure. But the perpetuation of the esoteric knowledge of the profession, and the transmission of the experience of practising physicians can only be seen to come about through the long medical training. One of the central features of this training is the clinical teaching, for it is here that the 'mystery' of clinical diagnosis is revealed.

Research in medical education, however, has rarely focused on the clinical context, perhaps because sociologists as well as doctors have readily accepted the belief that the processes involved are unavailable to documentation. Happily for us, the two following papers in the volume avoid this pitfall. In 'The Reproduction of Medical Knowledge' Atkinson discusses the nature of clinical teaching, and the symbolic significance of its place at the patient's bedside. To an outsider, clinical teaching may appear composed of casual, almost random discussions of a medical problem. Atkinson shows that this is not so. He documents the highly structured situation which is created for teaching, mirroring hospital practice only in certain features. Further, he emphasises the sharp control over the knowledge transmitted at this stage in the students' careers. In learning to become practising physicians, students must learn clinical skills through diagnosis. But as beginners, they can only handle the simple, the certain. The teaching is organised to withhold the uncertainties.

This paper, then, deals with the perpetuation of medical knowledge by discussing the clinical teaching which takes place at one point in the student's career. But the work also has implications that concern the perpetuation of the medical profession. For Atkinson draws attention to the 'clinical gaze', and argues for the centrality of this belief in medicine today. Such a belief provides a strong element of indeterminacy for practitioners, which affords them much of the privilege and status of their present position. To understand medicine, then, one must comprehend the nature of clinical practice. This paper offers us an aid to such comprehension.

M.R.

THE REPRODUCTION OF MEDICAL KNOWLEDGE

Paul Atkinson

The Bedside as a Field of Experience

As Foucault points out, modern medicine fixes its own emergence within a period at the end of the eighteenth and the beginning of the nineteenth centuries.[1] It was at this time that the modern 'clinic' was born — a distinctive combination of hospital teaching, a new mode of medical discourse, new methods of inquiry and so on. The 'clinic' has profound mythological significance for the profession of medicine. It provides the rationale for its empiricism, and a profound faith in the primacy of first-hand experience and perception at the patient's bedside:

> Medicine has tended, since the eighteenth century to recount its own history as if the patient's bedside had always been a place of constant, stable experience, in contrast to theories and systems which had been in perpetual change and masked beneath their speculation the purity of clinical evidence.[2]

It was therefore in the clinic that the prime justification of modern medicine evolved — in the directly perceived reality of the patient and the manifestations of his illness. Beneath the 'gaze' of the physician the superstructures of elaborate and abstract theories fell away. What lay revealed to scrutiny was the pure and uncontaminated perception of the individual patient and his illness. Or such soon became the mythological charter of modern medicine, at any rate:

> Clinical experience ... was soon taken as a simple, unconceptualised confrontation of a gaze and a face, or a glance and a silent body; a sort of contact prior to all discourse, free of all the burdens of language, by which two living individuals are 'trapped' in a common, but non-reciprocal situation.[3]

As Foucault describes it, the clinic was born in a radical reorganisation of medical discourse. Previous theorising had allowed for the classification of disease in systems which were ungrounded in the individual organs of the body. The clinic emerged when it became possible to treat the individual as a field of investigation, and that space by the patient's bedside therefore became the locus of medical inquiry and research, as well as treatment and instruction.[4]

Jamous and Peloille[5] have also commented on the emergence of the 'clinic' and its development in the nineteenth century. In common with Foucault they describe the unique combination of roles of teacher, researcher and clinician within the university hospital of the time.[6] During the earlier part of the century, hospital wards were the main research environment, as well as the locale for the instruction of apprentices to the practice of medicine. Jamous and Peloille go on to argue that in the course of the century, this unique combination fragmented. With the emergence of research in the laboratory the clinical practitioner lost his monopoly over medical knowledge and research. The researchers in the medical sciences were usually not those with access to the privileged positions in the university hospitals, and within the medical profession there developed a struggle for supremacy between the elite clinicians and the clinical and paraclinical researchers. A lengthy discussion of Jamous and Peloille is not possible here.[7] But one of their main points is relevant. They describe how the hospital clinicians sought, with considerable success to retain their social and professional superiority by an appeal to their pretheoretical clinical experience, and the privileged knowledge granted them by their clinical 'gaze'.

The nature of 'clinical experience' took on an elaborate set of connotations. The 'reality' of the bedside became arcane, and the clinicians' social and professional exclusiveness became matched by what passed for a privileged perception. The 'gaze' of the clinic became associated with a 'vision', which was treated as a personal quality ('virtuality' as Jamous and Peloille put it) of the practitioner. The clinicians therefore affirmed their privilege and status by virtue of the primacy of 'clinical experience' and the importance of bedside teaching in the transmission of such esoteric knowledge. They made great play of the 'indeterminacy' of core areas of knowledge and perception, and hence the importance of the apprenticeship mode of instruction and recruitment to the profession.[8]

With minor modifications, the account Jamous and Peloille offer can be generalised to cover the development of modern medicine in many contexts. Despite the fragmentation of medical knowledge and teaching, 'the clinic' and bedside teaching have retained their central importance. Throughout the changes in theory and practice in medical education, the clinical component has remained, in essence, unaltered at its heart. Its justification remains that which Foucault identified for the earlier epoch — an appeal to direct, pre-theoretical experience, which is taken to be antecedent to scientific theorising. Thus Foucault quotes a modern author:

> In order to be able to offer each of our patients a course of treatment perfectly adapted to his illness and to himself, we try to obtain a complete, objective idea of his case; we gather together in a file of his own all the information we have about him. We 'observe' him in the same way that we observe the stars or a laboratory experiment.[9]

Rather more prosaically, two American authors express the justification for clinical instruction:

> The student on the ward learns through actual experience and practice the role and functions of a physician as well as the nature, manifestations, and treatment of disease. He learns something of how illness and hospitalization affect patients and their families ... Above all, he learns how the physician makes observations and how he collects, records and analyzes the information obtained from the patient, the family and the laboratory.[10]

If the clinic was born in the period described by Foucault, then it is also re-born each day in the medical schools and their hospitals. The everyday teaching practices of clinicians in the hospital wards ensure this daily 'renaissance de la clinique'. At patients' bedsides the 'clinic' is reproduced and its mode of discourse is transmitted. Clinical medicine and clinical instruction thus recapitulate their own development and their own mythological past.

It was, and is, in the clinic that medicine finds its warrant in the privileged perception of the patient and his illness. Whatever the changing fashions of theory and treatment, there remains for medicine the pre-theoretical, pure experience of the clinic. Clinical work and bedside teaching provide the milieu in which the components of medical training are fused. They provide the combination of 'theory' and 'practice', of 'science' and 'practical experience' which are together taken to be necessary for the production of a competent practitioner.

To be sure, clinical teaching is by no means carried out solely by means of the traditional techniques. Nowadays it is supplemented by a wide range of audio-visual aids, simulation techniques and so on. Nevertheless, many of these are themselves reproductions of the bedside experience: bedside work remains the unquestioned guarantee of a stock of authentic medical experience in the training of a doctor.

In other words, in the world of medicine and medical education, competence is warranted by reference to a stock of 'experience' which has been acquired in the context of 'real medical work'. The primacy of this first-hand experience has been noted elsewhere. Becker and his co-authors[11] note the importance of 'experience' to students and teachers alike; they too take note of the connotations of immediacy and actuality in the reference to 'experience' by staff and students. In describing the 'clinical experience' perspective, Becker and his colleagues take it to refer to 'actual experience in dealing with patients and disease . . .'. It is used to contrast with 'theoretical' and 'scientific' knowledge:

> . . . even though it substitutes for scientifically verified knowledge, it can be used to legitimate a choice of procedures for a patient's treatment and can even be used to rule out use of some procedures which have been scientifically established.[12]

These authors go on to comment that 'argument from experience was quite commonly used and considered unanswerable'. Such unanswerable experience is gained in the context of clinical instruction — which is itself unquestionable.

Despite its central place in medical education, and its mythic significance for the medical profession, the topic of clinical bedside teaching has remained almost entirely neglected as a topic of research, both by sociologists and those practically engaged in medical education.[13] Consider, for instance, the Report of the Royal Commission on Medical Education.[14] In the course of this major review of undergraduate and postgraduate medical training, little attention is paid to the topic of bedside teaching; no radical evaluation of the teaching methods involved is attempted or proposed. The authors of the Report content themselves with a few paragraphs addressed primarily to the ethics of such teaching practices.[15] One's impression on reading the Report is that the theme of clinical instruction was almost totally taken for granted by the Royal Commissioners. The place of such teaching in the major clinical specialities is certainly not treated as problematic — for instance, the importance of clinical work and

The Reproduction of Medical Knowledge

experience in medicine and surgery. These are, traditionally, the two clinical specialities in which the students' initial experience of the 'clinical' is gained; their pride of place in the undergraduate curriculum has tended to go unquestioned.[16]

To be fair to the Royal Commissioners there was precious little published research that they could have drawn on in their deliberations. Despite the vast amount of available material in the general area of medical education, bedside teaching has been very poorly served. In one recent review of the literature[17] the lack of references to clinical teaching — in comparison, say, with those on selection and assessment procedures — is revealing. There has been a small output of observational studies of bedside teaching — based upon observation schedules and time sampling methods — but in the main these are woefully inadequate.[18]

It is common to assume that the sociology of medical education is ideally catered for, in so far as we have had major studies by Merton et al.,[19] Becker et al.[20] and Bloom[21] — the first two now treated as classics in the field. Certainly some aspects of medical education and student life are excellently documented and discussed in these studies. Yet, like their counterparts from 'inside' medical education, these studies signally fail to examine in any detail the nature of student patient interaction in the context of clinical teaching. (This is particularly striking in the case of *Boys in White*; here, if anywhere, one might have expected such ethnographic detail. Yet the authors even managed to omit the students' first contact and experience with patients altogether![22])

For members of the medical profession and for sociologists alike, then, the nature of the 'clinic' in medical education has escaped close scrutiny. Whilst its importance has been affirmed, its nature and conduct have remained unexamined. To some extent this can be understood as a reflection of the dominant styles of sociological research — especially in the field of education. It has only been with the emergence of the so-called 'new sociology of education' that the management of knowledge in educational settings has been a normal topic for inquiry.[23]

I strongly suspect, however, that there is a more significant reason for the neglect of bedside teaching in the major hospital specialties. It lies in the nature of the enterprise itself, and the nature of its taken-for-granted legitimacy. I refer to the fact that it is taken to depend on medical students' direct, personal exposure to the 'reality' of medical practice. Their first-hand experience of life and work in the hospital wards, clinics, operating theatres and so on, may appear to need little further elaboration. At first sight it may seem self-evident and natural that students should learn by being immersed in the real work of competent practitioners in their 'real-life' work settings. Just as bedside work provides a historical justification for the medical enterprise, so it has a self-justificatory air in its day-to-day practice. The world of medical 'reality' is taken self-evidently to furnish experience that the practitioner can rely on; he puts his trust in the evidence of his own senses and so amasses a personal stock of relevant knowledge. As Crooks[24] has recently expressed it, the outcome of this is that bedside teaching is 'an area which has tended to be "taboo" in curricula development'. He was certainly correct to identify clinical teaching as 'taboo', and the word is well chosen. It has connotations of the sacred — of 'mysteries' which only the initiated may glimpse or participate in, and an aura of such mystique surrounds clinical medical instruction.[25] The 'lesson of the hospitals'[26] is recapitulated every day. Yet it remains stubbornly invisible.

The Lesson of the Hospital

My own research in this area has been directed towards the day-to-day practices of bedside teaching — how the 'lesson of the hospitals' is taught and learned, and how 'the clinic' is reproduced.[27] The research was conducted by means of participant observation over two years in the Edinburgh Medical School. The Edinburgh Medical School — while by no means untouched by innovatory movements — preserves the tradition of clinical studies. Hitherto, the procedures of clinical teaching have remained relatively unscathed — a quiet eye in the centre of storms of change. To that extent, the research reported here may be thought of, in part, as itself a contribution to the 'archaeology of knowledge'.[28]

The bedside teaching to be discussed here is encountered in the students' first year of clinical work. The Edinburgh Medical School preserves the pattern of a segment of 'preclinical' studies, followed by 'clinical' years. It is in the fourth year of the course that clinical work is undertaken for the first time.[29] During this first clinical year the students receive instruction in general medicine and surgery, as well as continuing work in medical sciences. Students are attached to a clinical firm for each term, in groups of between eight and a dozen ('cliniques'). For the first term of the year all students attend medical units; in the second, one medical firm and one surgical firm.

The clinical teaching which is under discussion here cannot be taken

The Reproduction of Medical Knowledge

as entirely 'typical' of British medical education. There has been, and still is, a difference in emphasis between the Scottish medical schools and their English counterparts (especially the London schools). Crooks summarises it neatly: 'In England the tendency has been to use the "apprenticeship" system, with the student "walking the wards", while in Scotland there has been an emphasis on small-group teaching at the bedside . . .'[30] Bedside teaching at Edinburgh therefore has a distinctive flavour — with stress placed on 'Socratic' teaching dialogues at the patient's bedside. (However, since we do not have readily comparable ethnography from any other British medical schools, it is impossible to tell just how distinctive Edinburgh really is in this regard.)

Although it is by no means the only clinical teaching that the students experience, in this paper I concentrate on 'bedside' teaching as such. This is one of the most characterstic aspects of educational practice in the hospital. A clinician takes a small group of students into the ward and teaches at the patient's bedside. He may spend all the time available with one patient, or conduct a 'round' — taking in a number of patients in succession. Bedside teaching provides opportunity for a number of topics to be worked on: students practise taking patients' histories and performing physical examinations; they attempt to formulate differential diagnoses on the basis of their 'findings'; physicians and surgeons themselves may demonstrate their skills in these areas to the students. The individual patient may also be used as a starting-point for more general discussions of pathology, treatment, clinical method and so on. I shall now discuss some of the basic features of the conduct of such 'small group teaching', and the nature of the 'medical reality' that is produced and reproduced in such encounters at patients' bedsides.

The first feature to be noted is the scenic and 'ecological' arrangement of bedside teaching. In so far as the teaching is located in a hospital setting, it partakes of the medical reality of that milieu. In the accomplishment of bedside interaction, the medical locale is largely pre-constituted for the clinicians and students. For instance, the presence of medical personnel — nurses, porters, patients, other doctors, physiotherapists and so on — promotes a definition of the situation as a medical one. Educational work on the wards takes place against a backcloth of the ongoing routine work of the ward; it takes place in the midst of the normal coming and going, and the busyness of weekday mornings in a teaching hospital.[31]

In this sense, then, there is no difficulty in seeing the process of clinical teaching as one of exposure to 'reality', or immersion in the 'real' world of medicine. But it is not as simple as this. Although the teaching takes place within the hospital ward, it is to some extent insulated from it, and although there is constant activity in the wards, it does not necessarily impinge on the bedside teaching as such. As it progresses, the teaching round seems almost completely isolated from the other goings-on in the ward. As the clinician and his students stop at each bed, they form an 'ecological huddle'; as it moves round the ward, forming and re-forming round each new patient, the group is enclosed by a relatively impermeable 'membrane'.[32] The physically invisible, but socially marked boundary which encloses the group is seldom invaded and it is a noticeable disruption of normal affairs if this should occur. The teaching round is therefore one of those gatherings for which, as Goffman notes, 'the setting follows along with the performers'.[33] In this respect the teaching session resembles the consultant's 'grand round' – a similarly sacred procession. However, unlike these other processions, the students' rounds are solely educational exercises. They are not therapeutic in intention, and the routine care of the patients is kept distinct from the teaching of junior clinical students.

The management of bedside teaching means that there is little or no occasion for the interaction of the junior students with nursing and other paramedical staff members. The direction of the students' work is almost exclusively towards those tasks that are normally taken to be the preserve of the medical profession themselves (history-taking, examination and diagnosis). The invisible 'membrane' does not extend to take in the tasks that are routinely shared with, or delegated to other ward personnel. The boundary maintenance of social interaction on the ward parallels the boundaries of the division of medical labour and of professional dominance.[34] Working rounds and teaching rounds are kept quite distinct, and any inadvertent confusion of the two is normally taken as occasion for apologetic repair work and explanation. In this sense, then, although bedside teaching is located in the 'real' world of medicine, teaching encounters are constructed in a way that separates them from much of the routine work in that context.

In contrast to the day-to-day management of the patient, and the observation of corresponding changes in the patient's condition, the bedside teaching session is typically episodic in character. The patient's hospital career will normally be under way by the time that he or she is visited by the teaching clinician and the members of the

The Reproduction of Medical Knowledge

'clinique'. During the teaching episode, the patient's career — the trajectory of the illness, the processes of diagnosis and so on — are recapitulated by the doctor and the students. Typically, the patients who are taught on have already passed through routine admission procedures. They will have been referred to the hospital department, have been seen in outpatient clinics, or have arrived as emergency admissions. They will normally have been at least differentially diagnosed, and management of some kind will usually have been initiated. In some cases, the diagnosis can be taken as definitive by the medical staff. In brief, they will have been inducted to the position of hospital patient, with an emergent or fixed diagnostic identity. These simple contingencies provide the background to much of the construction of management of bedside teaching encounters.

The previous medical work that has been done on patients guarantees the 'medical reality' that is being enacted. (Amongst other things, it would distinguish it from simulation exercises using actors and role-playing techniques.) But if the bedside teaching is to provide a plausible and convincing re-enactment of 'real' medicine, this work has to be set aside. It is precisely this process of diagnosis that must be recapitulated in the teaching period, and the encounter therefore often proceeds on the unspoken assumption that such diagnosis has not in fact been done. Although the patient may have gone through his or her history on several previous occasions, students are routinely required to take a history 'from scratch', as it were, without reference to the production of these previous accounts. Students, patients and doctors all normally respect the rule that the previous medical work should not be directly referred to in the normal course of history-taking, examination and diagnosis.[35] The patient's part in preserving this aspect of the exercise may be crucial to its successful joint production.

It is possible that the patient may have become aware of the nature of his or her condition. But clearly such information should not be divulged by the patient prematurely — before or during the students' inquiries and speculations. For this to occur would undermine the validity of the history-taking exercise. Whilst this normally appears to be a rule that 'goes without saying', clinicians may at times explicitly guard against the patient spoiling the interaction in this way. Patients may be coached in being good subjects for bedside teaching. This can be illustrated briefly from the following extract from my field notes:

> The first patient Dr Potter took us to see was in one of the female wards ... Dr Potter asked her if we could look at her 'tummy'. She pulled up her nightdress to reveal a band of sore places round her midriff. Dr Potter asked Peter Bell, 'What do you think that is?' Turning to the patient, he added, 'Don't tell him what it is.'
>
> Peter Bell looked at her in silence for some moments, then said, 'She may as well tell me what it is.'
>
> Dr Potter hinted, 'Remember — the accent is on neurology.'
>
> 'Herpes zoster,' volunteered one of the other students.
>
> 'Herpes zoster,' repeated Dr Potter approvingly.

Now this is obviously a very abbreviated diagnostic exercise, which depended solely on the students' observation of the patient's 'tummy'; on this occasion the students were not required to take a history. Nevertheless it does illustrate how the patient's knowledge of her condition (and hence of previous diagnosis) is held in abeyance. And when students are taking a history, then patients are much more at risk of 'giving the game away' — in reply, perhaps, to the standard opening gambit of 'Could you tell us in your own words what it was that brought you into hospital?'.

The field-note extract can also be used to illustrate a further feature of such interactions (again in an abbreviated form). It is apparent how the previous work that has been done on the patient provides a resource for the teaching clinician. By virtue of his previous acquaintance with the patient, and the medical work that has been done on her, it is possible for him to direct the students' inquiries if the desired response is not forthcoming. In this example, his prompting, '... the accent is on neurology' elicits the missing 'diagnosis'. In this way the clinician is able to monitor the exchange of information between the patient and the students: he may do his best to hold back information from appearing too early, and facilitate its appearance if it is not forthcoming in the usual way.[36]

A further point can also be illustrated from this short fragment of data. The physician's prior knowledge of the patient and her condition allows him to be extremely *selective* in his approach to the teaching. In this example, the 'history' as such was absent: the students were required only to make one observation and to identify the condition on that basis alone. Once more, it is the resource of the previous diagnostic work carried out on the patient which provides for this practice. In this instance, it allows the teaching consultant to set up a display of the potential use of bedside *observation* as a diagnostic technique.

What I have been illustrating by reference to this single extract from my observations is the way in which the successful management of bedside teaching can depend upon the clinician's control over the prior medical knowledge available about the patient's condition. On this basis the doctor can: (i) select patients who will reliably display certain selected signs or symptoms; (ii) monitor and manage the flow of relevant clinical information between the patient and the students; (iii) conduct the encounter in such a way as to ensure the appearance of diagnostic information. Hence, in the course of their bedside inquiries, the students may be led towards the production of warranted diagnostic ascriptions.

These points can be illustrated further by reference to the following extracts from a transcript of bedside teaching. (Portions of the interaction are summarised in order to save space.)

> One student has been taking a history from the patient. He elicits this past history:
>
> *Pt:* Well, for over a year I've been bothered with pains in my stomach and I went along to my doctor and complained about it. He sent me up to the Eastern Hospital about six months ago for an x-ray on my stomach. I went up and it showed a small ulcer in my stomach and ever since that I've been bothered with the pain in my stomach ever since that and it's got — seemed to get — worse and worse and I — it — the only time it really bothers me is before my meals. I get a pain across my stomach and when I do eat it seems to settle it and it comes and goes at each mealtime.
>
> The student asks a number of further questions concerning the stomach pain. The consultant breaks in:
>
> *Cons:* Okay, fair enough. Now I would like you in turn to ask relevant questions — one question each — trying to get further into his history. And I think it is only fair to say that so far you have not elicited all the main symptoms. What other questions are you going to ask? You know, this is not the diffuse interrogation of what we have now got . . .

We can note at this stage how the previous diagnosis informs this latter comment of the consultant's. His remark that there remains further relevant information that the student has not yet elicited depends upon his knowledge of some previously established set of symptoms that *have* been discovered. (Such indications may have been established by the doctor himself, or by a colleague; the information will normally be available for such interpretation in the folder of case notes about the patient.) Hence the consultant can direct and prompt the students' inquiries towards the 'discovery' of these established symptoms as the outcome of their questioning. On the basis of the consultant's directive, the students variously take up the questioning:

Despite the fact that the doctor has proffered his piece of advice, the students' collective questioning does not, apparently, produce any information which is recognised as the missing symptom(s). The consultant breaks in once more, and now directs his attention to the patient:

St: Is there anything else that you feel – symptoms that you get with this pain?
Pt: No, it's just the pain I feel. That's all, nothing else.
Cons: Is that actually strictly true? You know, is there anything – I think the question really is – is there anything which is happening recently?
Pt: Well apart from the pain I seem to have been drinking, likes of water, milk, things like that. Because of this I seem to go to the toilet a lot more than I used to . . .

This last utterance of the patient was taken to provide significant new information: further questioning from the students (and prompting from the consultant) led to the diagnosis of diabetes in addition to the gastric ulcer. At this point the consultant can be heard as turning his management of the interaction towards the elicitation of the elusive further symptom – the patient's thirst. On the basis of his own knowledge of the patient's condition and history, the consultant is able to re-phrase the student's question so as to draw out the missing response. Thus he is able to preserve the purpose and intent of students' history-taking, by ensuring that the relevant information in fact appears as it should, and when it should.

Once more, in examining these extracts I am trying to illustrate how the bedside teaching encounter may be managed: how the available diagnostic information can be selected and organised by the teaching clinician in the course of his exchanges with patients and students. This organisation is done in such a way that the bedside session is enacted as a plausible and lifelike account of 'real' medical work. Students can therefore be required to embark on the process of inquiry and diagnosis, and the clinician can be confident that it will yield predictable outcomes. In this way the students are likely to 'discover' what they should 'discover', and the procedures of clinical inquiry are validated by the orderly appearance of clinical 'facts'.[37]

One further aspect of the students' 'discoveries' can be noted at this stage. The starting-point of their inquiries is usually not 'is this patient ill?', but rather 'what is wrong with the patient?'. As I have already indicated, the patients who are seen on the wards have already gone through the admission process, in the course of which a strong supposition, if not moral certainty, of illness will have been arrived at by the hospital personnel. The patients will warrantably be treated as 'ill'. Hence it is a reasonable and practical assumption for students to adopt that the patients are indeed 'ill'. This is, therefore, a basic decision-rule that the students can work with, and the assumption of illness is a very strong one in this context. At an early stage in their medical careers, then, students may learn the rationality of what Freidson calls the 'bias towards illness',[38] which appears to be a general decision-rule of medicine.[39] Such an orientation in the case of medical students is not simply geared towards being 'on the safe side', nor is it attributable to the enthusiasms engendered by passing fads and fashions.[40] For them, the assumption of illness is an entirely rational and practical orientation, and it is daily confirmed by their own 'discoveries' and the evidence of their own senses.

If we take this last observation with my previous remarks on the conduct of clinical teaching, then the implications of my argument can now be summarised. Although it takes place within the social and physical context of hospital life, the 'reality' of bedside teaching is a carefully managed version of medical work. By virtue of the features I have outlined, the students' investigations proceed on the assumption that identifiable disease is indeed present. Clinicians are able to monitor and control student-patient exchange in such a way as to ensure that relevant signs and symptoms are forthcoming, in accordance with the rules of bedside discourse and clinical inquiry. In the following section of this paper this line of argument is developed further.

Training for Dogmatism

The practice of 'guided discovery' in students' diagnoses is a version of what Bernstein has referred to as 'invisible pedagogy'.[41] The distinction which Bernstein draws between 'visible' and 'invisible' pedagogies rests on the manner in which cultural transmission and reproduction are accomplished: 'The more implicit the manner of transmission ... the more invisble the pedagogy'. Bernstein's arguments are formulated primarily in connection with varieties of pre-school and infant schooling, but *mutatis mutandis* they can be extended. Thus one of the characteristics of 'invisible pedagogy' that Bernstein isolates is that 'ideally, the teacher arranges the *context* which the child is expected to re-arrange and explore'. This facet of invisible pedagogy can quite clearly be recognised in the innovatory approaches of 'guided discovery' science in the secondary school, and in medical students' 'discoveries' of clinical diagnoses.

It is in the nature of 'invisible' pedagogies that the methods of social control should be 'transparent': in other words, the social mechanisms of knowledge production and transmission should not themselves be made apparent or explicit. Hence the organisation and construction of legitimised knowledge passes for an organisation that is inherent in the phenomena of the 'real world' under exploration and investigation. The knowledge of clinical medicine therefore passes for something revealed to the 'gaze' of the bedside student, and the invisible pedagogy of bedside teaching practices provide a device for the affirmation of the preconstituted nature of illness as an ontological entity.

Secondly, the suppression of the patient's potential understanding of his or her own condition, and the experience of his or her hospital career, is also significant. This reproduces a version of medical relationships and medical decision-making which parallel those noted by Bloor and Horobin.[42] They highlight how, in seeking medical advice, the would-be patient must, to some extent, act as a 'well-informed citizen' in evaluating the nature and gravity of his perceived symptoms, and in taking the appropriate action. Having been admitted to the position of 'sick person', the patient is subsequently required to adopt a role more closely akin to that of the 'man-in-the-street'.[43] Many patients in the teaching hospital are in the position of being 'well-informed'. But their own information and understanding is not routinely used as a resource in the conduct of bedside teaching: indeed its appearance can prove quite disrupting to the entire exercise.[44] The particular version of medicine which is reproduced on such occasions thus recapitulates the passive and subordinate position of the patient as a prerequisite to the display of expertise on the part of the students and their teachers.

In the course of this paper I have deliberately used the word 'reproduction' in two senses. First I have tried to indicate some of the routine practices whereby medical knowledge is transmitted in the medical school, and how, in the course of such transmission, medical culture is handed on from generation to generation. Secondly, I am arguing that this is accomplished through the enactment of *versions* of medical work. That is, bedside teaching encounters are constructed in such a way as to 'reproduce' selected features of clinical work, and thus to furnish warranted accounts of the patient's illness, hospital career and so on.

Elsewhere Sara Delamont and I have argued that such situations can be usefully paralleled by a consideration of 'guided discovery' science teaching at secondary school level.[45] We suggest that such teaching methods have distinct characteristics (shared with a variety of similar approaches). These methods of instruction depend upon the production of 'reality-like' contexts and tasks. Goffman has commented on such techniques:

> In our society, and possibly in all others, capacity to bring off an activity as one wants to . . . is very often developed through a kind of utilitarian makebelieve. The purpose of this practising is to give the neophyte experience in performing under conditions in which . . . (it is felt) no actual engagement with the world is allowed, events having been 'decoupled' from their usual embedment in consequentiality.[46]

In this context Goffman in fact cites a particular variety of medical reproduction — that of the mechanical simulation of patients and illness conditions.[47] Such clinical simulation represents a further degree of abstraction from 'real life', in so far as the patient is totally substituted for by the machine or manikin. To that extent, the bedside teaching that I have described does provide the neophyte with 'actual engagement with the world'. But as I have also indicated, the reality which is encountered has been 'decoupled'; it too is a version which reproduces selected features of medical work.

What is under consideration, then, is a variety of carefully managed and contrived situations which embody reproductions or 'replicas' of what are taken to be crucial features of real working situations. The pedagogical success of such encounters depends upon a degree of verisimilitude; their success also depends upon sufficient management and transformation of 'reality' so that orderly and predictable outcomes may be ensured.

Occasions of this sort are like 'working models' of the real thing. As such they may be compared with what Garfinkel and Sacks call 'mock-ups'.[48] They describe how such models may be used to render features of the world reproduceable, observable and teachable. In short, such 'glossing devices' render aspects of the world *tractable*. They select out certain features and certain relationships, but place them in an unreal or false context. Yet it is the very falsification of some of the conditions that allows for the manipulation and comprehension of the particular elements that are reproduced.

What is of interest is how these 'replicas' in educational contexts provide occasions for the *methodic* production of 'facts' and knowledge. What is at stake in the course of bedside teaching is that students should 'go through the motions' of diagnosis. In other words, the encounter is not managed simply in order to provide a *display* of the patient and his case. As I have already argued, the success of the exercise depends upon the *retrieval* of relevant information, just as it would be done under 'normal' circumstances, in 'real' medical contexts. The suppression of prior information about the patient, and the clinician's control of the situation serve to ensure that there should be an *orderly* production of knowledge in accordance with the appropriate procedures of clinical medicine.

Finally, I wish to touch on an additional feature in connection with the students' experience of medical 'reality'. So far I have dealt primarily with the creation and maintenance of a version of the medical world. I should now like to turn to the notion of 'experience' once more, in the light of my introductory remarks to this paper, and the intervening discussion. The rhetoric and ideology of clinical medicine run somewhat as follows. Although the clinical world may appear to be open to the inquiring gaze of the clinician, knowledge of the world of medicine must be painstakingly acquired by long exposure to that world. First-hand experience must be built up in the development of the practitioner's biography. Jamous and Peloille point out how the accumulation of such 'personal' knowledge is of central importance in the definition of professional competence and expertise. Direct exposure to 'reality' in the 'clinic' provides the practitioner with the warrant of such personal knowledge. Such expertise is held to inform the practitioner's actions in applying the

The Reproduction of Medical Knowledge

rules of diagnosis and care: it is a prerequisite to the competent use of such methods in actual settings.

There is no conflict between the apparent nature of 'reality' and such a view of 'personal knowledge'. On the contrary, it is the first which is held to warrant and validate the latter. Such conflict that is apparent is rather seen to be between 'reality' and 'theory' or 'fashion' — versions of knowledge and opinion which can, as it were, break adrift from their moorings in the practitioner's direct experience of clinical phenomena.

The importance of personal knowledge has, of course, been noted before — often in connection with the constellation of factors referred to as 'uncertainty'. Freidson provides a classic formulation. In his discussion of the 'clinical mentality', he draws on the evidence of *Boys in White*, on 'experience', and then continues:

> ... the practitioner is very prone to emphasize the idea of *indeterminacy or uncertainty*, not the idea of regularity or of lawful, scientific behaviour. Whether or not that idea faithfully represents actual deficiencies in available knowledge or technique it does provide the practitioner with a psychological ground from which to justify his pragmatic emphasis on firsthand experience.[49]

Here Freidson emphasises uncertainty of knowledge, suggesting that personal knowledge and experience are to be contrasted with notions of regularity and predictability. He also tends to account for this at the level of the psychology of the individual practitioner. Fox takes a similar view in her discussion of 'training for uncertainty', and like Freidson, she tends to treat it as a psychological problem that medical students need to come to terms with. In both classic discussions of the clinical mentality 'training for uncertainty' has been over-stressed: 'training for dogmatism' has been almost entirely overlooked.

'Dogmatism' is in no way the opposite of personal knowledge; it is part and parcel of the same view of 'experience'. The clinician who appeals to his personal knowledge does so not by reference to his uncertainty, nor necessarily to the uncertainty of his colleagues. Rather, he bases his actions and decisions on the unquestionable bedrock — the *certainty* — of direct experience. The clinician's justification is that referred to by Foucault, and it can be paraphrased thus: ' ... the patient's bedside has always been a place of constant, stable experience, in contrast to theories and systems, which have been in perpetual change and have masked beneath their speculation the purity of clinical evidence.' Hence the appeal to experience *is* taken to provide knowledge of regularity and stability; but this order is taken to be inherent in the phenomena, and open to the clinical 'gaze', rather than residing in systems of theory and fashion. The 'clinic' is therefore taken to provide the incontrovertible demonstrations of reality, in the direct perception of its regularities. The clinician is not therefore operating in a state of 'uncertainty', but rather operating on the 'sure' warrant of his stock of experience.

In this way, the student's exposure to the 'real' world of medicine reproduces the certainty and dogmatism of personal experience. As a matter of fact, Fox does make passing reference to such certitude in her paper, but it is noteworthy that this aspect of her work has been largely overlooked in subsequent commentary, and it is quite overshadowed by the emphasis placed on 'uncertainty'. Fox points out that students who are embarking on their clinical work find a degree of certainty in this context of practical 'reality'.

> In the atmosphere of the 'clinical situation', a student can feel his medical knowledge take root. The 'chance to see many of the things he has read about' reinforces what he has previously learned; and the fact that 'there is a patient lying there in the bed' proves to him that what he is currently learning is 'really important'.

In this context the management of clinical teaching can engender certainty, especially during the first year of clinical studies:

> It results . . . from the fact that in the third year he is relatively insulated from some of the diagnostic and therapeutic uncertainties he will encounter later. For one thing, the acute illness he sees on the wards and the explicit problems he handles in the clinics are often 'classic' or so manifest that he says they seem almost 'obvious' to him.

At this point Fox comes closest to a recognition of 'training for dogmatism', but the argument is not developed further along these lines.

In just the same way as described by Fox, the clinical teaching for junior students that I have been describing makes 'obvious' and 'explicit' the manifestations of illness. Hence the conduct of clinical instruction constantly reaffirms the certainty of personal knowledge, and the primacy of bedside experience in warranting medical knowledge.

The Reproduction of Medical Knowledge

Summary

In this concluding section I shall try to draw together the threads of the preceding sections. I have tried to indicate that clinical instruction at the patient's bedside is guided by the rationale that trainees should learn through some direct exposure to the 'reality' of practical work. This underlies the history, ideology and practice of bedside teaching. But in the course of bedside teaching it is rather a 'version' or 'working model' of such a presumed 'reality' that is enacted at the bedside. Such reproduction of medical work ensures that the methods of clinical inquiry reliably produce 'the facts of the case'; such 'facts' are in turn warranted by the methods of their production and reproduction.

The orderly and methodic production of clinical facts, and hence of 'illness', therefore suggests a rather different way of conceptualising the role of 'personal experience' in medical education. Hitherto it has been suggested that the major outcome of exposure to medical 'reality' is the so-called 'problem of uncertainty': that the certainties of the preclinical sciences give way to the ambiguities of diagnosis and uncertainty in the prediction of clinical outcomes. I do not seek to deny that 'clinical experience' carries such connotations. Clinicians make frequent appeals to varieties of tacit knowledge, and acknowledge that their information and skills are limited. But I argue that undue emphasis has been placed on such aspects of medical knowledge and that the reverse side of the coin – the certainty and dogmatism of personal experience – have received insufficient attention. Personal experience is used to warrant a stock of knowledge and action in which the clinician places his trust. It can act as the touchstone by which novel events and theories are evaluated. The 'working models' of medicine that are constructed at the bedside can therefore be seen as devices for the reproduction of medical certainty.

The practices of bedside teaching also recapitulate the structured inequalities of medical work – between doctors and other health workers, and between doctors and their patients. Illness is constructed in terms of the exclusive expertise of the medical profession. The methods of bedside instruction tend to preclude the negotiation of illness and health between the doctor and his patient, or the doctor and 'paramedical' personnel. Whilst students may encounter alternative conceptualizations of doctor-patient interaction and of interprofessional relationships in other contexts, the model which is embodied in the initial phases of clinical work is potent and enduring in the students' socialisation.

In conclusion it must be emphasised once more that this paper is based in part on intensive fieldwork in one medical school. We still lack adequate research on most aspects of medical education in Britain, and on bedside teaching anywhere. No exaggerated claims for 'typicality' and universality are intended in this paper; it is offered as a starting-point, rather than the final word on the matter.

Acknowledgements

I should like to thank Professor Liam Hudson and Peter Sheldrake, of the Centre for Research in the Educational Sciences, University of Edinburgh, for their support, encouragement and advice. My research in the medical school was made possible by Professor A. S. Duncan and Professor H. J. Walton, as well as the staff and students who bore my presence with great good humour. My ideas in this area have been clarified in my conversations with Sara Delamont, Margaret Reid, Anne Murcott and Rita Austin. The responsibility for this paper, with all its shortcomings, however, remains mine alone.

Notes

1. Michel Foucault, *The Birth of the Clinic* (London, Tavistock, 1973).
2. Ibid., p. 54.
3. Ibid., pp. xiv-xv.
4. Ibid., p. xiv.
5. H. Jamous and B. Peloille, 'Professions or Self-Perpetuating Systems? Changes in the French University Hospital System', in J. A. Jackson (ed.), *Professions and Professionalization* (Cambridge, University Press, 1970).
6. The university hospital as such pre-dates the emergence of 'the clinic'. What Foucault describes as the 'old clinic' must be dated back to the first half of the eighteenth century – to such institutions as Boerhaave's clinic at Leyden, and the early medical school at Edinburgh, founded on the Leyden model.
7. An extended commentary on their paper is contained in P. A. Atkinson, M. E. Reid and P. F. Sheldrake, 'Medical Mystique: Indeterminacy and Professional Process', Occasional Paper No. 14, Centre for Research in the Educational Sciences (University of Edinburgh, 1973).
8. The argument hinges on a distinction between 'indeterminate' and 'technical' means of production and reproduction. Jamous and Peloille attempt to use the notion of a ratio of indeterminacy to technicality as a way of categorizing occupations. Whilst their overall approach seems limited, the themes of indeterminacy and technicality recur in the ideological contests of professionalism and segmentation. See Atkinson *et al.*, for a development of this line of reasoning.
9. J.-Ch. Sournia, *Logique et Morale du Diagnostique*, cited by Foucault, p. xv.
10. G. L. Engel and W. L. Morgan, *Interviewing the Patient* (London, Saunders, 1973), p. 7.

11. H. S. Becker, B. Geer, E. C. Hughes and A. L. Strauss, *Boys in White* (Chicago, University Press, 1961).
12. Ibid., p. 225.
13. D. M. Levine *et al.*, 'Trends in Medical Education Research: Past, Present and Future', *Journal of Medical Education*, 49, February 1974, pp. 129-36. They note as one major lacuna in the research literature 'the microdynamics of student-faculty-patient interaction in the medical school'.
14. *Royal Commission on Medical Education* 1965-68, Cmnd, 3569 (London, HMSO), 1968.
15. Ibid., paras. 287-93.
16. There is of course nothing inherent in these areas which makes them the only conceivable candidates for such a place in the curriculum.
17. M. A. Simpson, *Medical Education: A Critical Approach* (London, Butterworth, 1972).
18. For a critical review of these studies, see P. A. Atkinson, 'In Cold Blood: Bedside Teaching in a Medical School'. in G. Chanan and S. Delamont (eds.), *Frontiers of Classroom Research* (Slough, National Foundation for Educational Research, 1975).
19. R. K. Merton, G. G. Reader, and P. L. Kendall (eds.), *The Student Physician* (Cambridge, Mass., Harvard University Press, 1957).
20. Becker *et al.*
21. S. W. Bloom, *The Medical School as a Social System. Milbank Memorial Fund Quarterly*, 49, 2, Part 2, 1971. Reprinted as *Power and Dissent in the Medical School* (New York, Free Press, 1973).
22. The initial exposure to such clinical work took place in the students' sophomore year. The authors believed that the student perspectives during that year would not differ significantly from those described for the years immediately preceding and following. They therefore paid little attention to this phase of the students' experience of medical school. (Becker *et al.*, p. 314.)
23. I refer primarily to developments outlined in M. F. D. Young (ed.), *Knowledge and Control* (London, Collier-MacMillan, 1971).
24. J. Crooks, 'Clinical Teaching in the Medical Curriculum of the University of Dundee', in *Curriculum Changes in United Kingdom Medical Schools* (Dundee, Association for the Study of Medical Education, 1975).
25. Cf. Atkinson *et al.*
26. M. Foucault, *op. cit.*, p. 64 ff.
27. This part of the paper is based upon completed participant observation research on clinical teaching in medicine and surgery in the Edinburgh medical school. I should like to record my thanks to all the staff and students there who made the research possible; my particular thanks go to Professor A. S. Duncan and Professor H. J. Walton for their support and encouragement.
28. When a great deal of activity and research is being devoted to the implementation and evaluation of *innovations*, it is all too easy to omit documentation of the 'old', the 'established' and the 'traditional'.
29. As in all Scottish medical schools there is a large intake into a first-year course in the basic sciences, so that many students have three years of preclinical studies, instead of the usual two.
30. Crooks.
31. The 'public' nature of such hospital life is emphasised by D. Gill and G. Horobin, 'Doctors, Patients and the State: Relationships and Decision-Making', *The Sociological Review*, 20, 4, pp. 505-20. On the importance of settings and personnel in the creation and maintenance of medical realities, see J. Emerson, 'Behavior in Private Places: Sustaining Definitions of

Reality in Gynaecological Examinations', in H. P. Dreitzel (ed.), *Recent Sociology No. 2: Patterns of Communicative Behaviour* (London, Collier-MacMillan, 1970).
32. Cf. E. Goffman, 'Fun in Games', in *Encounters: Two Studies in the Sociology of Interaction* (Indianapolis, Bobbs Merrill, 1961).
33. E. Goffman, *The Presentation of Self in Everyday Life* (New York, Doubleday, 1959).
34. E. Freidson, *Professional Dominance* (New York, Atherton, 1970).
35. This rule does not appear to be one in which students and patients are necessarily coached explicitly: but breaches of it are recognisably problematic and disruptive events.
36. This point is elaborated further in Atkinson.
37. This is discussed more fully in P. A. Atkinson and S. Delamont, 'Mock-Ups and Cock-Ups: The Stage Management of Guided Discovery Instruction', in P. E. Woods and M. Hammersley (eds.), *School Experience* (London, Croom Helm, 1976).
38. Freidson, *Profession of Medicine*, (New York Dodd Mead, 1970), p. 255 ff.
39. T. Scheff, 'Decision Rules and Types of Error and their Consequences in Medical Diagnosis', *Behavioral Science*, 8 (1963), 97-107.
40. Such fashions contribute, for instance, to the over-production of diagnoses of specific conditions (e.g., the fads for tonsillectomy – see M. Bloor, 'Bishop Berkeley and the Adenotonsillectomy Enigma', *Sociology*, 10, 1 (1976), pp. 43-62.
41. B. Bernstein, 'Class Pedagogies Visible and Invisible', *Class, Codes and Control Vol. 3* (London. Routledge & Kegan Paul, 1975).
42. M. Bloor and G. Horobin. 'Conflict and Conflict Resolution in Doctor/Patient Interactions', in C. Cox and A. Mead (eds.), *A Sociology of Medical Practice* (London, Collier-Macmillan, 1975).
43. A. Schutz, 'The Well-Informed Citizen, an Essay on the Social Distribution of Knowledge', *Collected Papers Vol. 2* (A. Broderson, ed.) (The Hague, Nijhoff, 1964).
44. Cf. Atkinson.
45. Atkinson and Delamont.
46. E. Goffman, *Frame Analysis* (Harmondsworth, Penguin, 1975), p. 59.
47. D. O. Levinson, 'Bedside Teaching', *The New Physician*, XIX (1970), p. 733.
48. H. Garfinkel and H. Sacks, 'On Formal Structures of Practical Actions', in H. C. McKinney and E. A. Tiryakian (eds.), *Theoretical Sociology: Perspectives and Developments* (New York, Appleton-Century-Crofts, 1970).
49. Freidson, *Profession of Medicine*, p. 169.

In the following paper Arnold Arluke discusses how the heart of the licence and mandate granted to the medical profession by society, lies in the assumption that the profession exercises control over the work of its practitioners. In recent years there has been an increase in the interest of both medical and government authorities in evaluating how the standards of health care are maintained. However, much of the subsequent research has focused on the statistical assessment of the indicators of the quality of care, rather than the nature and substance of social control by practitioners in their actual professional work settings.

In contrast to this typical research Arluke examines the mortality conferences of three teaching hospitals in the eastern sea-board of the United States. Mortality conferences are the occasions on which the death of patients are reviewed. It has been proposed that the death of a patient contributes perhaps the greatest threat to the medical profession, since such an event may not only throw doubt on the competence of medical practitioners, but also undermine the claim of the profession to control the work of its practitioners. Arluke therefore explores the mortality conferences to see how the problem of a death is managed, and to what extent the situation constitutes a machinery of supervision within the profession.

It is discovered, however, that the review of 'how a patient died' by hospital staff rarely becomes an arena of self-criticism and professional supervision. Through the routine methods whereby the mortality conferences are organised, the review of death becomes merely an academic exercise, with the emphasis placed on the educational aspects of the case at hand, rather than professional control of the work of practitioners. The issue of responsibility for the death is removed from the stage, and in so doing the importance of the death is defused. In the words of the author, 'the finger of blame is not only blunted but non-existent'. Occasions which contain the potential of undermining the professional worth are so organised that the professional collective remains unchallenged. The author likens the situation to one in which primitive people reassert their social solidarity through ritual, and in so doing establish routines to manage the problem.

C.H.

SOCIAL CONTROL RITUALS IN MEDICINE:
The Case of Death Rounds*

Arnold Arluke

Professions or key occupations claim to possess competence over a body of knowledge and a collection of techniques. These claims can be seen as a form of myth-building, explaining to participants and to the general public what typical members of a profession do, how they do it, why it needs to be done, and how capable they are of doing their work. To the extent that others believe these claims and trust that there is no serious disparity between professional promise and performance, responsibilities will be awarded to the profession.[1] An essential component of these claims to trust is that the professionals themselves are both willing and able to regulate the current competence and performance of practitioners. The exercise of social control by the profession over its members is thought to ensure that the gap between professional promise and performance does not usually occur, and when it does occur, is not serious. The assumption of effective social control, therefore, lies at the core of professional authority.[2]

In the case of the health sector, both medical and government authorities have been increasingly concerned with means of assuring reasonable standards in the provision of medical care and in evaluating the delivery of health care in settings where teaching as well as treatment are carried out. However, the literature on evaluating systems of health care delivery in hospitals almost always focuses on indicators of quality of care, including the composition and outcome of various hospital review committees, hospital mortality rates, utilisation rates, credentials of medical staff and so on.[3] Virtually no attention is directed to the actual practice of medicine in the hospital and how regulation and control of professional performance in that setting is accomplished.[4] Until the time health services research refocuses its efforts on the processes of social control, the claim of the medical profession to exercise effective internal peer review of performance will remain unsubstantiated.

In a general sense, any attempt to regulate medical performance has

This research was financed by United States Public Health Service Grant No. 5, Pol H S 00013.

within it the potential for a professional emergency. The evaluation of professional work poses a risk to individual practitioners and the general profession of identifying mistakes and questioning competence. Each profession has its own way of managing emergencies and coping with errors and possibly mismanaged situations. Indeed, the social organisation of professional work is constructed around mistakes and situations where mistakes may surface.[5] As Hughes notes, relations among members of a role set are partly organised, 'to delegate, to spread, or in some cases, to concentrate the risk and guilt of mistakes; and also to spread and allocate losses which result from them'.[6] Devices that serve the latent function of transforming professional emergencies into professional routines are, in their most rudimentary form, a legitimising apparatus or social control ritual.[7] In his study of the Andaman Islanders, Radcliffe-Brown suggests certain rituals in medicine may produce 'a condition in which the unity, harmony and concord of the community are at a maximum, and in which they are intensely felt by every member'.[8] Rituals will emerge in professional settings to normalise mistakes and routines that could otherwise become a professional emergency. The deviance-reducing features of social control rituals in medicine deserve further attention.

Perhaps the greatest professional emergency in medicine is the death of a patient. Although death is a recognised risk, its finality arouses strong feelings, especially among physicians in training.[9] Unlike other medical events, death can challenge the efficacy of the individual practitioner as well as the profession as a whole. A death resulting from professional error not only questions the competence of those responsible, but casts doubt on the profession for not having exercised sufficient supervision and control in the first place. In the professions, mistakes are as much a commentary on those who make them as they are on those who permit them. Patently, the review of death is an inherently problematic event for the medical profession; the possibility of mistake or error cannot be ignored.

In teaching hospitals, the principal device for scrutinising the deaths of patients is the mortality review conference, referred to by the medical staff as 'death rounds'. These conferences are not explicitly viewed as a supervisory mechanism; rather, their primary purpose is believed to be instructional. However, in the academic milieu of teaching hospitals it is difficult empirically to separate the concepts of supervision and education. The exercise of supervision and the process of instruction are thought to occur simultaneously.[10] From such a perspective, death rounds are seen by the medical staff as ultimately functioning in a social control capacity even though they are formally designated as a teaching conference. The fact that death rounds are designed to exert control indirectly through the process of instruction and teaching does not necessarily mean that control will be exerted at all, or if exerted, that it will be effective. This paper[11] will explore the supervisory and instructional processes of death rounds and examine the nature and substance of social control in this setting.

The analysis which follows is based on observations of thirty-two death rounds, representing over sixty cases reviewed. The field work was conducted in three different teaching hospitals along the eastern sea-board of the United States. The hospitals are all large, prestigious university-affiliated institutions servicing major metropolitan areas. More selective and focused data were collected by interviewing and interacting with members of the medical, surgical, pathological and radiological staffs of these hospitals. These included forty-five lengthy interviews with interns, residents, and attending physicians. Interview and observational work was directed by the general concern of this research with the problems of social control in the context of professional training.

Of course, much of this research was based on observational data and is thereby subject to all the biases inherent in such data. In order to cope with the problem of selective observation, attempts were made to keep complete records of all that transpired during the death rounds observed. Observations eventually reported were cross-checked between individuals and between various modes of observations as well as with the interview data. There is no intent to suggest that the death rounds studied are representative of any larger universe of professional medical conferences in other services or hospitals. However, in so far as some of the attributes of these rounds are generated by the hospitals' commitment to the training, education, and control of physicians, similar characteristics may be encountered in the review committees of other institutions and services. Comparison of the findings made in this report with previous studies of professional behavior in hospital settings indicates that the social organisation of the hospitals studied is comparable to that of other teaching hospitals affiliated with universities.

The Dramaturgy of Death Rounds

Internal medicine death rounds are a weekly, one-hour conference, devoted to analysis and discussion of the deaths of two ward patients. Attendance is open to anyone, although attending physicians, residents

Social Control Rituals in Medicine 111

and interns from medicine and medical students compose the bulk of the audience. Staff members start to filter into the conference room ten to fifteen minutes before death rounds actually begin. Routinely meeting in one location gives staff members an opportunity to talk about a variety of concerns ranging from problem patients to house staff parties. These informal pre-conference gatherings also provide the staff with a chance to talk about death rounds themselves. One can occasionally overhear, for instance, a group of interns and residents discussing a case presented at one of the previous death rounds, commenting on particular features of the presentation that interested them.[12]

Formally, death rounds begin with a general introduction by the moderator of the two cases to be presented. Following the moderator's brief description of the cases, an intern or resident from internal medicine presents the first case. The presentation includes summaries and interpretations made by the presenter from the patient's chart, including admission complaint(s), pertinent medical history, social history, results of physical examination on admission, results of examinations and tests, treatments and medications administered, and the hospital course of the patient, culminating, invariably, in death. Providing information relevant to the patient's subsequent death, from the perspective of an observer, has the appearance of an orderly and literal reading of the chart. A resident comments on this appearance:

> Usually there is very little editorializing that goes on in determining what to present and what not to present. I mean, there really aren't significant editorial changes in the content of the chart. You present the salient features of the case. And usually that's adequate and it isn't misleading. (5. Resident)

The matter-of-factness of presentations is one of the most prominent features of death rounds, one to which staff members orientate and seek to preserve.[13] This orientation is apparent in discussions by the staff of the quality of presentations.

A 'good' presentation at death rounds, according to the staff, summarises all the pertinent information in the chart in under five minutes. The presentation is delivered to the audience without pause in a manner that permits the listener 'to get a picture of what went on with the case'. The presentation must convey a 'feeling' for the case:

In a bad presentation you don't bring out the relevant data. And you bring out extraneous information making it unclear exactly what happened. In a good presentation, you can sit down, hear the presentation, and have a good feeling for what happened. You know what happened chronologically. You don't have many questions and blank spots as to what really happened. (17. Intern)

In addition, the presenter must not only recreate a sense of clinical presence for listening physicians, but must also be prepared to answer certain questions about the case. He may be asked, for example, to provide special details about a particular test given to the patient or he may be asked to postulate about underlying disease processes in the case.

Presentations are generally stylised in a way that suggests the presenter is so familiar with the case that he could have been the patient's primary physician, even though he was not. This effect is achieved in several ways: the presenter can occasionally refer to a few, sparse notes; he can glance through the patient's chart and construct the presentation as he moves along; or there can be no reliance on charts or notes. His pauses are rare, he uses test results sparingly, but selectively, creating a rising crescendo of medical events that ends dramatically with the patient's death, 'even though we did everything we could for the patient'. The image created by the presentation is of a patient who has been 'run through' all the usual procedures, thereby demonstrating that the medical staff has done its job, sufficiently for all practical purposes.[14] The orderly execution of presentations at death rounds achieves the desired outcome; the medical staff is seen as having done its best — death could not have been avoided.

The routine of death rounds can be depicted as a series of presentations or steps.[15] Radiologic findings normally follow the initial presentations made by interns and residents. As with the opening presentations, radiologic presentations are also from the pre-mortem perspective. By displaying numerous X-rays, the radiologist indicates how diagnostic decisions were arrived at in the case under discussion. The X-rays are shown in the same chronological sequence in which they were originally taken. Ostensibly, his presentation is an attempt to document visually the clinical course of the patient. The radiologist's remarks tend to buttress comments made earlier by others at death rounds and leave the audience feeling that the diagnosis and treatment are acceptable. What others can do only with words, the radiologist can do more convincingly with 'hard' visual data. It is not uncommon

Social Control Rituals in Medicine

in the course of the radiologist's presentation to observe several physicians leaving their seats and walking up to the X-rays to inspect them more carefully and to express their interest and curiosity in the films. Responses such as these from the audience do not dispute the radiologist's interpretation; rather, such actions guarantee a normal and ongoing course of affairs at death rounds. Once completed the radiologist's presentation sets the stage for the pathologist.

Usually given by a resident, the pathologist's presentation is organised around a series of slides shown in rapid sequence. Most of the slides feature individual body organs photographically captured to display the pathology detected at autopsy. Frequent microscopic sections of tissue complement the gross descriptions. As each slide appears on a large screen in front of the audience. the pathologist identifies and discusses the particular pathology. His talk, however, is an interpretation of what is going on in diseased and normal tissue and is an opinion based on an evaluation of what he sees. Generally, the pathologist's manner and tone are understated, but declarative and firm. The 'guessing game' quality of death rounds seems to disappear as the matter-of-factness of the pathologist's report proceeds. Some staff members characterise the pathologist as a 'heavy':

> Some pathologists play the part of the heavy. It's not so much showmanship and flair, but it's sounding like . . . It's putting together the events that occurred in a pathophysiologic sense in a way that's understandable, rather than just to say, 'Well, the liver section showed this, and the lung section showed this . . . and so the diagnosis is this.' Flair is when they can draw together and they can follow the patient's clinical course and put in the pathologic information that kind of solidifies their description of the pathologic course. (29. Intern)

The work of assembling clinical clues and correlating them with pathological findings usually results in a final diagnosis and occasionally a different perspective on what the best course of treatment might have been for the patient. Even in those cases where the pathologist is unable to state an exact diagnosis or cause of death,[16] he is still seen as having the last word:

> He's considered to have particular insight. He's got the final word. It's very difficult to refute the pathologist unless you're debating his pathological findings. And in order to do that with any kind of

credibility you have to be a pathologist, although that's not entirely true. If you're a gastroenterologist and you know quite a bit about liver pathology, you could probably question him on a liver section. If you have special expertise, you can debate with the pathologist. But as a general internist, you're not going to debate with him much at all about very specific pathologic evidence. (4. Intern)

The Routinisation of Death Review

Although they are referred to as death rounds, there is typically little discussion of death at these conferences. The importance of death is de-emphasised by concentrating the work of review on the pre-mortem course of patients. Of course the staff knows that the presentations conclude with death. But death becomes more of a vehicle for noting the progress of the conference than a central organising device for conducting review. Death is simply not 'dealt with' from any perspective at death rounds:

> In the sense that mortality conferences deal with death, death isn't that important. They don't deal with death as a rule. They don't deal with death philosophically. Death isn't dealt with as anything, but that's the end of the meeting. Death is a misnomer. They really focus on the clinical course and clinical problem. (13. Resident)

The significance of death is diminished by directing instructional interest on the events that lead up to death. The medical staff believes that physicians can learn more from the circumstances that precede death than they can from the death itself. Consequently, what makes death rounds unique as review conferences is not the matter of death; rather, it is the realism and detail of the cases presented. This 'realism' is thought to make death rounds particularly instructive for the staff, as an intern points out:

> What's special about death rounds is having one or two patients discussed in great detail and having everything reviewed. The setting is very realistic because the case is not sterile.
> Somebody in the room probably had a lot to do with it. The rounds are special in that sense . . . and that's what makes them fairly instructive. Whether or not the patient even died . . . that doesn't mean much educationally. (40. Intern)

While an attempt is usually made to connect the pre-mortem course of patients to their death, this connection is often done in a cursory manner. Indeed, the link between post-mortem and pre-mortem circumstances, as well as the more general relationship between patient and disease, are not seen as crucial links to the learning process at death rounds:

> If it's a patient you didn't have responsibility for and that is getting presented as a case, it's just that. The case is being presented. It is not a patient that you know and whose death might hold some personal significance for you. What is being presented is a disease, its complications, and its course. That's what is educational. You're not looking at death and you don't think about what patient it was. I mean, these things don't effect what you learn. (14. Intern)

To many staff members, death holds little 'interest'. What is interesting for them at death rounds are the unusual physiological complications and clinical problems of some patients. Obviously, not all deaths will pose interesting pre-mortem circumstances for the staff. Cases that are uninteresting are not viewed as good cases for instruction and are therefore not presented at death rounds. The more complex the patient's medical history and professional management, the greater the chance it will be seen by most staff members as an interesting case and, of course, a good teaching case. One of the residents in internal medicine describes an interesting case as follows:

> Usually the interesting thing about a case is what nature does, not so much the actual death. Like just having many complications occur over time. Having the patient respond in an unpredictable way, or not responding to therapy. Or having a complex and somewhat bizarre set of clinical problems. (9. Resident)

Another resident says:

> Interesting and instructive cases are not your everyday common deaths. If it is an everyday common kind, there's something about it which makes it instructive. Generally, it's a case that has been either a very sticky diagnostic problem or therapeutic problem. It may also be a case in which the diagnosis was not arrived at before death. Some cases are interesting because several different therapeutic programs were used and none of them worked until a certain time, and maybe one of them worked, maybe none of them worked. Something about the case that makes it complex also makes it interesting. (22. Resident)

'Complex' cases demonstrate the many different problems that physicians in clinical practice can face. It is the concentration of a variety of problems in a single case that makes it unusual and interesting for the staff, as is illustrated in an example below:

> I remember one complex case. The patient was in the hospital for a long time and developed all kinds of complications. And many people in the hospital saw this patient at some point. He was somebody who got shot in the leg. Had to have his leg amputated. I think he might have been shot in the abdomen too. And he developed all kinds of complications ... He developed respiratory failure. He developed adrenal insufficiency. He developed multiple infections ... psychological problems ... He was reviewed in great detail. He had some very complex problems. And he was probably in the hospital for six months. He was in the hospital for most of my internship year. And he came in the hospital shortly after I got here. So all the interns knew him. You know, in everyday practice you'd never see a patients like this. This wouldn't occur over the span of a hundred patients. (12. Resident)

It is the very compactness of a wide range of problems into one case that makes it valuable as a learning experience for the medical staff. Reliance is placed on physicians to conduct their own learning, testing themselves any time they feel ready during death rounds. The test is self-scoring and self-interpreting. However, by choosing cases that have a high concentration of problems and by relying on staff members to test themselves, there is no guarantee that they will learn from all or even many of the problems posed during death rounds. In so far as complex cases have an instructional value, that value may well be lost:

> It's up to those present to make it an exercise in going through the logical processes of coming up with a diagnosis and treatment plan and seeing the experience of individuals involved with the patient and the successes and failures they had. You don't have to make a personal declaration as to how you would have handled the case. You just ignore the autopsy findings and try to abstract yourself clinically from the case. Sure, some aspects will interest me more than they will somebody else. But most everyone will find something about the case that interests them and when they do, that's when they're likely to test themselves. (30. Resident)

Whether or not an individual physician tests himself is a decision left entirely to the discretion of each staff member. If he decides to test himself on a particular feature of a case, the evaluation does not depend on arriving at the final diagnosis or matching the most appropriate treatment plan suggested in the course of death rounds. Should a discrepancy exist between the staff member's own thinking and that of his colleagues, it is not problematic. Testing in the instructional setting of death rounds, refers to the exercise of clinical judgment more than the correctness of that judgement. The sheer complexity of the cases being discussed directs testing toward the process of clinical judgement rather than its outcome. Certainly, staff members point out alternatives to the care and management of patients; indeed, these alternatives may imply that a mistake may have been made. Yet, it is difficult to view a particular decision as incorrect in a setting where discussion about judgement reduces to an equivocality:

> Frequently people will disagree with a number of things that were done on the care of a patient. And this may imply that they think a mistake may have been made . . . they would have done it differently. But people don't call these differences mistakes because it's very uncommon that a decision is so obviously wrong that a person could be justified in saying that kind of thing. Usually there's some argument for what the person decided to do, therapeutically or diagnostically. If you should call something a mistake, you're very likely to be refuted. There just are not very many truths that you can say and be absolutely on solid ground. How can something be a mistake if it's a controversial point in the first place? (18. Resident)

Complex cases inevitably involve complications and 'extenuating circumstances', making the assessment of outcome an inherently problematic task. One of the residents elaborates this point in the following quotation:

> I don't think certainty is high enough so that really black and white criticism can be made very often. But when it is, it's still difficult to call something a mistake because when something goes wrong, and there's a hint that there has been a blunder, there are also other extenuating circumstances. There are other complications that have happened concurrently and you're not sure what was the cause of death. It's almost never clear, in the

kind of cases we get at death rounds, that somebody made an error that just isn't excusable. (24. Resident)

By inspecting clinical judgement in light of subsequent events, professional decisions are assessed as part of an unfolding pattern of what 'all along' had been a complex and demanding case.[17] As a practical feature of the work of reviewing death at death rounds, physicians understand discrete decisions made early in the course of patient care in the context of what is now known about the case. What could be seen as an inappropriate decision or mistake becomes, by the end of the conference, a reasonable judgement for any practitioner in those circumstances. In the words of one of the second year residents:

As things unfold it becomes clear that a decision made way back in the course of the patient may not have been the best decision, even though the majority of those sitting in the room clearly would have done the same thing were they handling the patient. The whole element of 'if such and such had been the case', the element of armchairing . . . I don't think that's a large part of death rounds. Usually such a statement is prefaced or ended by, 'Of course, none of us in the room would have thought to do that'. There isn't justification for being critical. The physician on the case ends up being in the minority at the end of the conference, even though most everyone at death rounds could imagine making the same decision he did at the beginning of the case. And when this happens it is instructive, and people are empathetic with the person who made the mistake . . . it is not even right to call it a mistake . . . it's a decision that turned out to be less than optimal. (11. Resident)

Under circumstances such as these, differences of opinion regarding the medical management of a case are seen as 'academic' differences that do not reflect on the competence of the responsible physicians. Physicians say that discussions of alternative approaches to cases are instructive and serve as a vehicle for learning something from what was done to the patient:

You'll see the infectious disease specialist and the oncologist stabbing daggers and throwing flaming swords at each other over some point made in the presentation. But it's all in the sense of academia and roundsmanship and that kind of interchange . . . One guy will cite some studies and talk about his clinical

Social Control Rituals in Medicine 119

experience to show that a test that wasn't done, should have been done. And we all learn from these interchanges. (6. Intern)

In fact, some staff members compare the nature of discussion at death rounds to the quality of conversation in a seminar:

> So people will say, 'This is the way I would have handled it. Why didn't you consider this?' Or, 'Did you consider this alternative?' If somebody raises a question like this, there's almost always more than one answer that is acceptable. In a way, it's like the conversation and discussion that you hear in a seminar or in a forum where papers are being presented. (16. Intern)

By pointing to the complexity of the case and orientating to the educational features of the discussion, errors become excusable and mistaken judgements become understandable. By invoking complexity as a descriptor of the case, those findings presented after the fact at death rounds do not transform a physician's earlier judgement into something that was inappropriate, given the circumstances faced by the physician at the time the decision was made. Mistakes are normalised in this context and become 'less than optimal' judgements that anyone present at death rounds might make were they in a similar situation. Emphasis on the instructional intent of death rounds effectively removes any real disapproval from the identificaiton of a mistake by stressing group learning over individual censuring.

As a major feature of the routine of death review, physicians hope that their colleagues will conduct themselves properly in this context and not disrupt the educational temper of the conference. A value is placed on comments at death rounds that are felt to be most instructive for those physicians in attendance. Indeed, particular staff members develop reputations for making intelligent contributions and promoting general education, as an intern remarks below:

> There are doctors here who are noted for being very good at death rounds. They make instructive and intelligent comments. They are facile with the literature. They make points that they don't have to back down from very often. They know what they're talking about . . . ah, you know, what they say is going to sink into plenty of us. (19. Intern)

Conversely, physicians who criticise individual colleagues for their management of a case are viewed as disrupting the ongoing instructional process of death rounds. These physicians risk being seen as unprofessional, especially if their criticism is direct, blunt, and 'unacademic'. The staff member who is 'tactless' at death rounds may face 'ostracism' by his colleagues for breaking the educational flow of discussion:[18]

> Some people make critical comments and they are less tactful than others. When they make a comment, it's taken in the context of the kind of personality they have. Nobody pays much attention to it. Criticism needs to be done in an academic way. Otherwise, it won't be very helpful. I mean, you don't see people standing up and saying, 'Well you idiot. Why and the hell did you do that for?' It just wouldn't happen. If it did happen, the person who stood up and said it would be ostracized. (20. Intern)

To avoid disruptions to the instructional routine of death rounds, steps are taken by the director of medical education and others before the rounds begin. Members of the medical staff believed to have been involved in making 'unwise' decisions are not selected to present their own case at death rounds. Were they to make such a presentation, it may appear as though they were being 'put on the spot'. A deliberate effort is made to minimise disruptions and control departures from the educational routine of death rounds by removing responsibility for patient care as an issue, as a member of the staff reflects below:

> Death rounds are a totally academic exercise and responsibility for patient care there is not in question. What we are taking is just a disease entity. The patient and his physician become separated from the disease. It doesn't matter what patient's name is attached to it. And it doesn't matter what physician took care of the patient. We're just discussing a specific patient, but he could belong to any physician as far as we're concerned. What's important there is the disease and the way you go about looking at it. (7. Attending)

In the following anecdote, a consultant speculates as to why he was selected to present a particular case at death rounds:

I presented one patient who had a spinal cord tumor and who had several complications. I can't say with complete confidence, but some of these complications probably could have been avoided. I had consulted on this patient. I was working with the hematology group and we consulted on this patient. When I presented it I wasn't any more nervous than if I were speaking to the Lady's Aid about the emergency services of the fire department. But I think if I were the doc who was primarily responsible for the care of this patient, in whom some very unwise decisions were made, I probably would have felt pretty uncomfortable. I presume that's why they picked me to present, because death rounds isn't a chopping block for the person who presents. That isn't the atmosphere. There may have been somebody involved . . . in fact, in this case where I was the consultant, there was some question about a couple of the decisions made. But the attempt is not to put someone on trial. The attempt is to avoid that. (28. Resident)

The selection process for choosing the presenters of cases at death rounds, according to respondents, reflects a general concern for maintaining a normal state of affairs during the conference. Furthermore, cases that portend 'troubles' difficult to contend with in light of the normal activities of death rounds may not come up for review at all. Should a case involve known 'blunders' and possible malpractice questions, it will not be selected for presentation:[19]

If there are some troubles with . . . if someone blew it and may even be responsible for malpractice . . . These kinds of cases do not come to death rounds. I think when bad blunders occur, there is some attempt to keep them quiet. And if they are kept quiet, they're not going to get to death rounds. (36. Resident)

From the point of view of the medical staff, careful selection of an appropriate physician to present a case and a suitable case to discuss is necessary to preserve the instructional intent of death rounds and to avoid confronting 'troublesome' issues. Without deliberately managing the organisation of the confernece, it is thought that the substance of review may go awry.

Pedagogy and the Possibility for Control

Malinowski[20] suggests that among groups of primitive people, death threatens social solidarity and activates expressions of defence. Cohesion is saved by making a social ritual out of the event of death.

Those who participate in a ritual become increasingly tolerant of undesirable events and behaviours. By constructing a ritual around problematic situations, the situation itself becomes embodied in a routine. In the profession of medicine, accounting for the event of death raises a risk of finding deficiencies in the individual practitioner and the profession. Death review is a highly precarious process; the underlying potential for review to cast doubt on the competence of physicians and the worth of medicine is considerable. Findings of this study suggest that the formal review of death in teaching hospitals manages this precariousness in such a way that professional worth is not challenged.

In order to establish a professional routine around the review of death, it is necessary effectively to diffuse the importance of death. By focusing on the clinical course of patients, death becomes a natural end to the review process. It is not death that is interesting to the staff, but rather the clinical complexity of the case. The work of review becomes an 'academic exercise' in assembling case histories out of disparate pieces of clinical evidence and impressions, invariably impressing those present. At the conclusion of the review, the main feeling is one of being impressed by the reviewers for their skills in conveying a 'feel' for cases. The reviewers imply that had anyone else managed the case, the patient's death would still not have been avoidable.

The matter-of-factness of death review is further enhanced by normalising the issue of mistakes and removing the matter of professional competence from the agenda. Deciding the appropriateness of professional judgement after the fact becomes a moot point given the complexity of the cases discussed. Fault is not placed on any individual physician. Indeed, responsibility is rarely even a peripheral issue at death rounds. The sense that any physician facing similar circumstances might warrantably do the same thing pervades the conference. The main theme of death rounds is the determination of how patients die clinically, not medically. The finger of blame is not only blunted but non-existent. In this context, talk about professional failure rather than biological failure threatens the routine of review. Efforts are taken to preserve this routine by managing the nature of cases presented and by separating responsibility for the case from the act of presenting it.

By reducing the significance of death and removing professional competence as an issue, the instructional intent of death rounds can proceed. It is difficult, however, to sustain belief in the stated purpose of death rounds — to achieve indirect social control over professional performance by pedagogy. The audience responds to many features of the review having little to do with serious instruction. The process of learning as well as the assessment of learning are left to the discretion of each physician. Lessons are not extracted from the discussion and communicated to those present. Individual cases at death rounds are not compared to previous cases, thus preventing the identification of patterns in patient care. In short, the process of instruction at death rounds seems to be a casual afterthought to the routine of review. Somehow learning is presumed to take place in this setting without ever having to specify what it is that should be learned. This analysis does not suggest that it is impossible for physicians to learn anything at death rounds. People do learn in real-life educational situations, but often what they learn are the attitudes and sensibilities needed to be accepted as a member of a particular group or community. In the case of death rounds, I argue, physicians may acquire a special conception of medical work and what constitutes its appropriate review. To the extent that review conferences such as death rounds successfully transmit such a conception of proper review, the likelihood of achieving indirect social control is reduced, if not precluded.

Notes

* Data presented in this paper are as they appear in the original field notes and interview transcripts. All quotations are identified by code number only.

1. William J. Goose, 'Community Within a Community: The Professions', *American Sociological Review*, 22 (1957), pp. 194-200.
2. For a recent attempt to conceptualise the issues involved in social control and its relationship to authority, see Sanford M. Dornbusch and W. Richard Scott, *Evaluation and the Exercise of Authority* (San Francisco, Jossey Bass Publishers, 1975).
3. Freidson writes, '... the danger of the future is that reliance on formal modes of administrative measurement will create a facade of accountability without providing any insight at all into the quality of health care.' (Eliot Freidson, 'The Development of Administrative Accountability in Health Services', *American Behavioral Scientist*, 19 (1976), p.296.)
4. This is with the exception of Freidson's analysis of social control in a group practice. See Eliot Freidson, *Doctoring Together: A Study of Professional Social Control* (New York, Elsevier, 1975).
5. See, for example, Donald W. Light, Jr., 'Psychiatry and Suicide: The Management of a Mistake', *American Journal of Sociology*, 77 (1972), pp.821-38; and Jeffrey W. Riemer, ' "Mistakes At Work" The Social Organization of Error in Building Construction Work', *Social Problems*, 23 (1976), pp.255-76.

6. Everett C. Hughes, *Men and Their Work* (Glencoe, The Free Press, 1958), p. 98.
7. For a more complete discussion of this point in the context of secondary socialisation, see Peter L. Berger and Thomas Luckmann, *The Social Construction of Reality* (New York, Doubleday, 1967), pp. 138-9.
8. A. R. Radcliffe-Brown, *The Andaman Islanders* (Glencoe. Ill., The Free Press, 1948), p. 252.
9. Joan Stelling and Rue Bucher, 'Vocabularies of Realism in Professional Socialisation', *Social Science and Medicine*, 7 (1973), pp. 661-75.
10. This idea was originally suggested to me by Mary E. W. Goss.
11. This research is drawn from a more extensive study that focused on the problems of social control in the context of professional training.
12. It can be argued that the formal framework of review conferences provides an occasion for informal social control to occur.
13. This analysis benefits from Zimmerman's research on the reception function and intake procedure in a public assistance office. See Don H. Zimmerman, 'The Practicalities of Rule Use', in Jack D. Douglas (ed.), *Understanding Everyday Life* (Chicago, Alsine, 1970), pp. 221-38.
14. Ibid., pp. 226-7.
15. These steps, from the vantage point of the medical staff, seem to progress in a 'realistic' sequence from admission findings to autopsy findings. The presentations of the internist, radiologist and pathologist appear to build on each other, making a continuous chronology out of a collection of often discontinuous circumstances.
16. Sometimes during death rounds it seems more important for some diagnosis and cause of death to be attributed to a patient, than none at all.
17. See Harold Garfinkel, *Studies in Ethnomethodology* (Englewood Cliffs, New Jersey, Prentice-Hall, 1967), chap. 3.
18. Such displays show an inadequate grasp of participants' shared understandings of proper action on a given occasion. Individuals who suspend the instructional routine of death rounds and raise the issue of competence may themselves be seen as incompetent. These breaks in routine serve as important learning devices for newcomers.
19. Goffman notes, 'It can be assumed that the possession of a discreditable secret failing takes on a deeper meaning when the persons to whom the individual has not yet revealed himself are not strangers to him but friends. Discovery prejudices not only the current social situation, but established relationships as well; not only the current image others present have of him, but also the one they will have in the future; not only appearances, but also reputation.' (Erving Goffman, *Stigma* (Englewood Cliffs, New Jersey, Prentice-Hall, 1963), p. 65.)
20. Bronislav Malinowski, 'Death and the Reintegration of the Group', in *Magic, Science and Religion* (New York, Doubleday, 1949), pp. 47-53.

References

Berger, Peter L. and Thomas Luckmann (1967), *The Social Construction of Reality* (New York, Doubleday).
Dornbusch, Sanford M. and Scott, W. Richard (1975), *Evaluation and the Exercise of Authority* (San Francisco, Jossey Bass Publishers).
Freidson, Eliot (1975), *Doctoring Together: A Study of Professional Social Control* (New York, Elsevier).
Freidson, Eliot (1976), 'The Development of Administrative Accountability in Health Services', *American Behavioral Scientist*, 19, pp. 286-98.

in Health Services', *American Behavioral Scientist*, 19, pp. 286-98.
Garfinkel, Harold (1967), *Studies in Ethnomethodology* (Englewood Cliffs, New Jersey, Prentice-Hall).
Good, William J. (1957), 'Community Within a Community: The Professions', *American Sociological Review*, 22, pp. 194-200.
Hughes, Everett C. (1958), *Men and Their Work* (Glencoe, The Free Press).
Light, Donald W., Jr. (1972), 'Psychiatry and Suicide: The Management of a Mistake', *American Journal of Sociology*, 77, pp. 821-38.
Malinowski, Bronislav (1949), 'Death and the Reintegration of the Group', in *Magic, Science and Religion* (New York, Doubleday).
Radcliffe-Brown, A. R. (1948), *The Andaman Islanders* (Glencoe, The Free Press).
Riemer, Jeffrey W. (1976), 'Mistakes At Work: The Social Organization of Error in Building Construction Work', *Social Problems*, 23, pp. 255-67.
Stelling, Joan and Bucher, Rue (1973), 'Vocabularies of Realism in Professional Socialization', *Social Science and Medicine*, 7, pp. 661-75.
Zimmerman, Don H. (1970), 'The Practicalities of Rule Use', in Jack D. Douglas (ed.), *Understanding Everyday Life* (Chicago, Aldine).

The traditional conception of the medical profession is of a collection of persons who, among other things, share a body of formally organised knowledge. Within this conception professional medical work is understood to involve the implementation, through the use of the scientific method, of schemes of interpretation found in the shared body of knowledge. Academically this conception has led to the suggestion that only those researchers who share this body of knowledge are able to examine or are justified in examining professional medical activity.

In the following paper Hughes examines the way the staff of a hospital casualty department categorise patients. This paper reveals how, on any occasion of applying medical knowledge to a case at hand, the staff unavoidably rely on their everyday knowledge of the world. In doing so, the professionals, rather than simply acting in accord with the strictures of scientific enquiry, also engage in practical or commonsense reasoning to make sense of the case and its circumstances. In this way medical decision-making can be seen to have many of the properties of decision-making in many everyday settings.

Rather, therefore, than being altogether hindered by a lack of specialised medical knowledge, the sociologist is able to provide insights into the socially organised character of the medical world. Consequently the possibility of intricate analysis of the social aspects of medical work is firmly placed on the agenda of medical sociology.

C.H.

EVERYDAY AND MEDICAL KNOWLEDGE IN CATEGORISING PATIENTS

David Hughes

The medical sociologist with an interest in the nature of day-to-day medical categorisation finds himself immediately confronted with the widely prevalent notion that the practice of medicine depends on the specialised knowledge of medical personnel. His colleagues concerned with the study of professions often mention such a body of knowledge as one of the prime attributes of any professional group,[1] and the recent Merrison Report (1975) provides an illustration of how medical administrators sometimes share this kind of idea, when it states that 'the essential character of a profession is that the members of it have specialised knowledge and skills which the public will wish to use'.

In this paper I neither seek to question the usefulness of the concept of specialised knowledge or to deny its importance for medical diagnostic work, but it does seem to me that sociological accounts of medical categorisation run the risk of oversimplification if they place central emphasis on formal training and technical expertise. For those of us who remain for most of the time remote from everyday medical work, there is sometimes a tendency to see medical categorisation as a largely unproblematic process in which determinable patient conditions are identified by procedures deriving from scientifically based knowledge — a view which may lead us to gloss over many of the practicalities of such work. Observational research which I undertook in a hospital casualty department[2] led me to believe that the categorisation of patients could be plausibly seen as a process of practical decision-making, which shares many of the features of everyday theorising in other settings. Stress on the importance of specialised knowledge often carries the implication of a sharper distinction between 'expert' and 'everyday' knowledge[3] than can plausibly be demonstrated to exist. As well as depending on specialised knowledge, the identification of patients' conditions depends on elements of knowledge which are presumed to be known to all, and indeed various elements of knowledge seem to merge in casualty staff's theorising in a way which can make retrospective distinction of specifically medical knowledge difficult.

Admittedly the very mention of 'everyday' as opposed to 'medical'

Everyday and Medical Knowledge in Categorising Patients 129

knowledge carries a certain risk of reification, but the distinction is implied in much everyday discussion about the work of the medical profession and is hard to avoid. On such grounds as that medical knowledge historically involves the elaboration of the everyday and that the boundaries remain unclear, a hard distinction is easily faulted. I do not offer the dichotomy between 'everyday' and 'medical' as a description of clear-cut substantive bodies of knowledge, but use the terms with the assumption that they bear some rough correspondence to distinctions made in everyday accounts. The general point is that knowledge conventionally labelled 'medical' is embedded in, and in certain senses dependent for its significance upon, the kind of knowledge usually thought of as 'common-sense'.

One feature of the casualty department which clearly illustrates the importance of everyday knowledge is the widespread involvement in the categorisation of patients of staff who lack significant formal training. Typically, those patients whose conditions are not straightforward to identify have a series of contacts with staff in which various definitions of their conditions may be advanced. Ambulance men, porters, and reception workers and even escorts or other patients can play important parts in labelling patients' conditions, in assessing the urgency of their need for treatment, and in bringing them to the attention of nurses and doctors. Often such early interactions will shape the form of the patient's subsequent passage through the unit and provide a framework of interpretation when more 'expert' personnel eventually encounter the patient.

Doctors are later likely to give importance to the accounts of such staff and to the account of the patient himself of the circumstances surrounding the case. This should alert us to the importance of 'what everybody knows' even in doctors' diagnostic work. While we may recognise the significance of medical expertise, we need to reflect carefully on how it is displayed in everyday interaction.

It could be said that practitioners' claims to medical expertise lie less in common access to a finite number of substantive elements of knowledge than in presumed familiarity with a more general shared perspective. Doctors assume that they share a grasp of professionally warranted schemes of interpretation. Within a general orientation they apply methods and procedures which allow certain determinable conditions and disease entities to be recurrently recognised in their patients. Yet, on-the-spot observation in any medical setting will indicate that use of such schemes of interpretation does not exhaust or adequately describe the practices that medical personnel employ to make categorisation decisions. Interpretative schemes made available by formal training may be used alongside or tend to merge into those made available by commonsense knowledge.

The perspective that I follow maintains that the sensible character of ongoing situations is largely dependent on the applicability, on each successive occasion, of typified knowledge of the dimensions of the social world. Staff members in the casualty setting experience their tasks as episodes in the mundane working day. Like anyone else they are continuously engaged in a task of making their environment meaningful and intelligible by ordering their experiences in terms of familiar categories. Outside of their working lives they construct definitions of situations and make identifications of objects and events in much the same way as others, and there are very many occasions when this ability is utilised in the practice of medical categorisation.

An obvious point is that the patient's condition often relates to events and objects that simply lie outside the scope of medical knowledge. Consider the following short excerpt from an unexceptional conversation. A man with a chest injury had just been brought in from an ambulance in a wheelchair.

> Ambulance attendant: 'He's been hit in the chest with a pole.'
> SEN: 'What kind of pole?'
> Attendant: 'A telegraph pole.'
> SEN: 'Has he? He'd better go on a stretcher then.'

Or take this extract from a conversation between a doctor and the escort of a man who had been 'hit on the head with a ball'.

> Doctor: 'Was he unconscious at all?'
> Escort: 'No.'
> Doctor: 'Was he dazed?'
> Escort: 'Not really.'
> Doctor: 'Was it a hard ball?'
> Escort: 'It was a golf ball. We were at the golf club.'
> Doctor: 'What time?'
> Escort: 'Seven-fifteen.'

In both cases staff members are able to draw on their everyday knowledge of what objects, telegraph poles and golf balls, are like and how they are likely to affect human bodies. No elaboration of the objects apart from general information about the balls and poles is asked for and the conversations move on.

Casualty staff encounter a constant succession of novel situations in which typified knowledge must be applied again and again to order and locate features of new scenes. Knowledge of typical actors, conditions, motives, courses of action, and matters of fact presumed in accounts commonly offered by staff members to explain patients' attendance is certainly not wholly medical. In many commonplace cases, for example, minor trauma, recognition is experienced as being immediate and almost automatic. In others it is far from straightforward. The mere arrival of a person at the casualty unit does not necessarily lead staff members to view him as a 'genuine' case. They recognise that people with no pathology are likely to present themselves for treatment and that sometimes the absence of pathology will be difficult to detect. They know that there are such types as malingerers, hypochondriacs, troublemakers, but identification of these types is not possible on strictly medical criteria. Negative findings on the small number of items in a typical examination would not conclusively rule out the possibility of a condition which might later be labelled illness. In these situations the ability of staff members to provide (for themselves and each other) an intelligible account of a person's presence seems to be the crucial factor in terminating or continuing the processing of the presenting patient. If a plausible account of why someone came to the department can be constructed there is no need for staff members to arrange anything more than routine checks. Consider the following case from my fieldnotes:

> (On Wednesday afternoon) Dr A, an Asian immigrant, was talking to an elderly man in the corridor. The man was noticeably unkempt. His clothes were old, and he was unshaven. I had noticed him sitting in the waiting room and he had now been called through. I did not know why Dr A came out of his room to question the man but he appeared to be having difficulty in determining the man's condition, and asked the man a number of rapid questions. 'What is wrong? . . . Why have you come here today? . . . Have you got a headache?' The man's answers were mumbled and inaudible. Dr A went away and eventually the man was taken to be examined by Dr B. I did not witness the examination. In the nurses' room a staff nurse was talking to another about the case and said that the man had fallen down and banged his head. Dr B came and joined the conversation, saying that she knew the man from previous

visits. 'He likes coming down to see us. He goes to have his hearing aid fixed and comes here as well. He's from ——— (old people's home).' The doctor repeated that she had seen the old man more than once, and said they would 'check his head' and give him some pills. The man was x-rayed and sent home.[5]

My interpretation of this case on my admittedly incomplete observations was that the man initially posed a classification problem. Staff members were faced with a man who could not communicate his condition adequately and knew only that he might have some kind of head injury. It was not a subsequent medical examination which resolved the problem, but Dr B's personal knowledge of the man as 'the old boy from ———'. Dr B's remark that the man 'goes to have his hearing aid fixed and comes here as well' seemed to carry the implication that it was not unusual for this particular individual to come to the unit and that no medical reason need be present for him to do so. I infer that this remark is embedded in typifications about the 'sort of things old people are likely to do'. The man was given routine medical examinations, but I would argue that this involved a 'check' on a decision already made, and represented the desire of staff members to 'cover' themselves. I observed many instances when uncertainty and even concern over the condition of newly arrived cases vanished when a staff member recognised a client from a past visit, and other staff members drew on their typified knowledge of the likely implications of the patient's status as a 'regular' to make the present visit understandable. A client will still be given certain basic examinations, but the urgency with which he is processed, the style in which he is handled, and the exhaustiveness of medical theorising, do seem to be influenced by the framework of expectation provided when such commonsense typifications are taken to provide plausible ways of seeing presenting patients.

Where there is uncertainty, questions such as 'why did he come then?' always seem to be raised, and theorising about the possibilities becomes a topic for all staff types. The precise character of accounts advanced to explain a patient's presence naturally depends on staff members' construction of the particular circumstances of the case, but a number of motives of causes are recurrently offered as possibilities.

Suggestions that psychiatric abnormality is involved are made quite frequently, but tend to blur with notions about the patient's social incompetence or moral culpability in a way which usually makes it difficult to describe them as unambiguously medical accounts. Staff members speak of patients as psychopaths, ex-mental cases, or psychotics without it being clear that they are not simply using such terms as general derogatory labels. It is common for mention of mental abnormality to be linked with mention that the person is nevertheless 'cunning', 'crafty', or has some rational end in mind. The following extract from my field-notes, for example, indicates how reception staff imputed a utilitarian motive to one psychiatric outpatient:

> (Friday afternoon.) The clerk indicated a card to me: 'Here's a social problem case. As far as I can gather he was down at the social security office. They wouldn't give him any benefit and he dialled 999. When the ambulance brought him up here he said that there was nothing wrong with him.'
> There were several record cards, including two treatments for overdoses, treatment for injuries arising from an assault, and various other minor injuries.
> Receptionist: 'First they thought the social worker has phoned to bring him in. But then it came out that he'd phoned himself.'
> Clerk: 'We think he perhaps wants a meal ticket.' She told me that the doctor had seen the boy and referred him to the local psychiatric hospital. He was an outpatient and had been due to attend for an appointment the following week. The clerk did not feel that this was useful: 'I don't see what they can do.'

The notion that patients who had no determinable physical pathology nevertheless stood to gain something from their attendance was present in much of the staff discussion of patients. Gaining overnight accommodation is an intention often ascribed to patients whom staff take to be without a permanent address. One doctor, for example, expressed the opinion that 'if we gave every psychopath in —— (town) a bed for the night we'd have no room for other people'. Coming to the hospital out of curiosity or in search of perverse self-gratification may also be mentioned. A porter told me, with some disgust, about persons who came 'for the day' and even brought sandwiches to eat in the outpatients' canteen. Speaking about 'malingerers' who came to the unit late at night a doctor told me:

> The ones who come here come for fun because they want to ride in an ambulance or because they want to get home. Usually it

is because they want to get home. They have been out. They have spent a couple of pounds on drink so they can't afford a taxi. They don't want to get a bus – all the buses have stopped – so they come here so they can have an ambulance.

Suspicions that patients are seeking drugs or attempting to escape the attention of other social control agencies by feigning illness also seem to have a commonsense quality, but come to figure in medical diagnosis from time to time. The points I have made have obvious relevance when non-illness definitions of patients' conditions are advanced, but in all types of cases staff draw on everyday knowledge to form a picture of what is before them. Staff must try to relate signs and verbal accounts, and place the presenting patient's condition in a context. Routinely nurses and doctors attempt to collect elements of information which will allow presently discernable features of the patient to be seen as the culmination of some understandable course of events, and when they are unable to do this they often become uneasy. On one occasion, for example, a Medical House Officer, who had been able to gather almost no information about an unconscious man taken off a train, stopped to talk to me about the case: 'It's the kind of excitement I don't want. I like to have a story. What was he doing on the train? Where's he come from? How did he collapse?' I said that I supposed in that kind of case doctors would have to concentrate on the physical signs. 'Yes,' he replied, 'but I'm afraid that you need a story to be able to interpret the physical signs.' A 'story' provides additional indicators which might document a particular underlying condition. The 'fit' of theorisations with the context outside of the patient's immediate appearance can be checked, and commonsense reasoning of the kind: 'If it was X then that would explain Y', can buttress diagnosis on clinical grounds. Often it is a feature of a scene which has meaning by virtue of commonsense knowledge which makes the pieces of a picture fall into place.

In a number of incidents that I witnessed the arrival of two apparently similar cases in a short space of time was itself taken as a clue to the likely conditions of the patients. An illustration is provided by a further extract from my field-notes:

(Wednesday night, 9.15 p.m.) A male in his late teens arrived in an ambulance with its beacon flashing. The attendant described the youth as a 'collapse', and said that the ambulance had been called by a girl who 'found him banging his head against a wall' in the street. The stretcher was wheeled into the corridor and an SRN, an SEN, the ambulance men, and several student nurses stood around apparently attempting to get a response from the boy by pinching his flesh, pulling his hair, and making remarks (in what struck me as a jocular manner) such as 'come on then wake up'. The boy appeared to be comatosed. His eyes were shut and he did not make any sounds, but he did move in response to the physical stimuli. Staff members seemed to view the situation with an attitude verging on amusement; they did not seem to view the case as 'serious'. The stretcher was pushed to the resuscitation room, but at that stage a staff nurse came from the nurses' room saying that she had just heard that a 'stabbing' was on the way in, and suggesting that the youth had better be moved to the recovery room as 'he looks alright'. I had the impression that the nursing staff were sure that he was responding correctly, although no specific suggestion of the nature of his condition was put forward at that stage.

Five minutes later another youth in his late teens was brought in from an ambulance in a wheelchair. Like the first youth he had long hair and was clad in denim jeans. The youth (whom I shall refer to as B in distinction to the first youth, A) seemed drowsy, and an SRN remarked that he seemed to be in a similar condition to A. She suggested that: 'Two is a bit too much of a coincidence . . . they must have taken something.' B was accompanied by another youth, and the SRN approached him and asked him what B had taken. He replied that he had found B 'staggering around' and had gone up to him because he 'vaguely' knew him. B had asked if he would take him home, but he couldn't walk properly and had fallen down and hit his head. He then called the ambulance. The staff nurse seemed to doubt the story, and she suggested that it would be for B's 'own good' if he told the truth. She took the escort to look at A to see if he knew him.

A was still in the recovery room, and an SEN was trying to wake him and examining his arms for injection marks. The Casualty Officer arrived to examine him and her immediate question about whether this was 'the drug case' led me to believe that the patient must have been mentioned to her in those terms. The SEN told her that there were two cases and that they seemed to have taken something together. The doctor said nothing during the examination and appeared to check the youth's chest, reflexes, and pupils. She mentioned that she thought it was drugs and left. I was able to get some idea of the doctor's view from the treatment card on which she had written that there was no sign of neurological damage, pupils respond equally, reacts to pain, and 'drugs'. A was then taken for a skull x-ray.

Without it being necessary to quote my notes about the further processing of the case, I think the importance of everyday knowledge in the recognition of the youth's condition as involving drugs is fairly obvious. My impression was that initially staff members had no clear idea about the youth's condition, but drew on their experience of the appearance of various conditions in deciding that there was no necessity to view the patient as a serious case. This was so despite the ambulance crew's use of the flashing beacon, which is usually taken to signify the seriousness of the incoming case. Possibly the information that the youth had been 'banging his head against a wall' led them to doubt the likelihood of a serious physical pathology being present. At that stage I could detect no sense of urgency or mention of bringing the case to the doctor's attention (although it was a quiet period and the doctor was not busy). The resuscitation room is simply the nearest room in which a stretcher can be put, and the move to the recovery room when a potentially serious case was expected reinforced my impression that the staff members were not concerned about the youth's condition. The arrival of the second youth in an apparently similar condition seemed to be the factor (perhaps taken together with the 'hippy' appearance of both youths) that suggested drug use. Notions about the limits of coincidence, types of people, and typical courses of action seem to derive from the SRN's everyday knowledge. She was able to suggest drugs as the explanation of the youth's condition by (to use Garfinkel's language [Garfinkel, 1967]) embedding the appearances in presupposed knowledge of social structures.

Another example involved a youth who had been brought by the police to the department, because of his bizarre behaviour following an incident in which he was said to have caused damage to a house and fought with police officers when they took him into custody. After remaining on a trolley in the recovery room for some time the youth made a sudden dash down the corridor towards the exit, but was caught by a policeman. His action seemed to be taken to indicate that his 'illness' had been a device to avoid custody, and he was immediately taken back to the police station.

Apart from the importance of commonsense typifications in understanding the circumstances of a case, many of the devices which staff members use to make a 'story' emerge, could be said to have been learned in the course of day-to day life. The logic and form of much of the decision-making that I observed would be apparent to individuals lacking medical training.

In everyday talk in the casualty department, staff can be heard engaged in such recognisable activities as asking questions, seeking elaboration, making assertions, and offering explanations. It is true that medical knowledge is associated with a technical language not familiar to most ordinary language users, but the talk of personnel in the casualty setting does not read like the printed texts that might be taken to characterise medical language. Styles of speech use vary considerably as different staff interact with patients at various stages of their passage, and as individuals attend to features of particular situations. A range of medical terms, colloquial expressions, and more everyday language is used as speakers vary language use in the light of the anticipated competence of their audience, or the direction and style of a particular conversation. Within the practical circumstances of casualty work seemingly adequate communication between staff about patients' conditions often proceeds without the use of technical medical terms.

Casualty staff's theorising typically lacks the rigorous logic and conscious concern over the adequacy of grounds for decisions that we might expect to find if medical categorisation could be characterised as a scientific activity. Staff are usually concerned with immediate priorities, the next step, rather than detailed determination of a patient's subsequent examination and treatment requirements. It is not uncommon, during the processing of less straightforward cases, for definitions of the patient's condition to change dramatically without any feeling among staff that anything exceptional has taken place. And because it can be seen that decisions are not taken on a once-and-for-all basis, it is quite usual to accept hypotheses about a patient on the basis of probable accuracy rather than conclusive determination. I mentioned that casualty staff are often faced with patients whose conditions cannot be ascertained with any certainty, but they still construct definitions which are adequate for the purposes of processing the patient. The general scheme available to practitioners on the basis of their medical knowledge needs to be applied to particular individuals in situations, and I would suggest that practitioners must use forms of *ad hoc* reasoning to facilitate this. Often the signs, symptoms and histories associated with particular cases are not available in an unambiguous form which readily articulates with formal medical knowledge to facilitate a diagnosis. Signs, symptoms and histories have to be assembled and arranged into a pattern, and the kinds of grounds taken to suggest a direction often have a commonsense quality. Many unexceptional staff practices illustrate this point. As in many areas of everyday life where previous contacts with individuals structure current attitudes towards them, past encounters with patients' conditions are taken to be a valid base for current hypotheses. One often hears remarks like 'I've seen him before and he's an epileptic', which are taken to justify treating the patient on the basis of the known condition. Another very common assumption in everyday reasoning is that location of objects in particular categories on the basis of observed features carries the implication of the presence of further unseen features which are known to characterise objects of that particular type. Such an assumption is often reflected in the direction of doctors' actions as they seek to locate signs and symptoms and reach some estimation of the relative plausibility of a number of possible conditions. As in most other reasoning processes, the apparent compatability and appropriateness of observed features, when they are viewed within some known frame of reference, is taken to establish relationships and the relevance of that framework. Concomitantly, if certain perceived features are inconsistent with claimed or hypothesised conditions, doubt about the presence of that condition is raised. Many of the elements of information relevant to a particular decision regarding the patient will have been derived from verbal exchanges, and as in many everyday life situations much will be taken for granted about the status of such accounts. When a staff member is introduced to a patient with a brief description from a colleague, he can only assume such things as the other's familiarity with relevant details of the case, that communicated information is well founded, and that particular procedures said to have been carried out have been performed competently. Often there will be no easy way of checking, and a staff member will have to draw on his own knowledge of usual organisational practice to decide what must have happened before he encountered the case. Patients' and escorts' accounts are usually likely to be given a similar importance. It is unexceptionally assumed that they attended to the events relating to their visit and will be able to provide relevant information although there will be no means of ensuring that they actually did so. Where there is scepticism about patients' accounts, it is usually because staff take as grounds for doubt such commonsense devices as attention to inconsistencies of claims, the existence of obvious utilitarian motives for lying, or the possession of a compromising case history.

I should emphasise that my mention of the importance of knowledge deriving from experience of everyday life for medical categorisation, does not in any sense imply a criticism of medical professionals. No suggestions that the kinds of everyday practices that I described imply a departure from some set of 'ideal' technically based procedures is intended. In my view any situation in which organisation members are required to process a client population is likely to be characterised by the kind of attention to typified knowledge and commonsense logic that I have tried to describe.

What the reported observations do perhaps support is the oft-made point that medical settings should not be seen as isolated scenes of social action. The formal training and even the informal organisational socialisation of personnel in the casualty setting do not negate the importance of cognitive resources made available by membership of a wider cultural formation in everyday definitional work. More open recognition of this rather innocuous point offers little real threat to the medical profession and may even have certain practical advantages. My own observations suggest that there is often a certain tension when staff, who routinely use the kinds of commonsense strategies that I have mentioned, feel obliged to offer a glossed account of their actions if their competence is at issue. One can occasionally detect a feeling among casualty staff that routine practices are departures from commonly accepted images of appropriate action, and that criticism could be expected if knowledge of how things 'really' got done became public. A more open acknowledgement of the mundane everyday features of medical practice (perhaps in medical training, at least) might remove some of this apparent guilt and uncertainty. It might similarly counter the unrealistically narrow view of the range of patient details that are legitimate medical concerns that pervades many discussions. More directly, recognition of the role of everyday knowledge in the practice of medicine has interesting implications for the currently topical communication problems of immigrant doctors. It might be that training programmes need to take account of the point that such doctors do not simply face a 'language problem' in a narrow sense; their problem is one of practising medicine in a situation where they lack the conventional knowledge available to most other participants.

Notes

1. Julius Roth mentions a number of writers who take an 'attribute' approach to the professions in his critical paper 'Professionalism: The Sociologists' Decoy' (Roth, 1974).
2. This paper reports one aspect of a research project that I carried out while I was the recipient of an SSRC studentship.
3. The suggestion that medical knowledge cannot be divorced from everyday knowledge has similarities with the notion that science, more generally, cannot be seen apart from commonsense knowledge and personal judgements. See, for example, Michael Polanyi (1958) and Henry C. Elliot (1974).
4. Some interesting insights into the part of non-medical staff in categorising patients in American Emergency Departments are contained in Julius Roth and Dorothy Douglas (1971) and David Sudnow (1967). This area deserves more study in Britain.
5. Passages described as extracts from my field-notes have been changed slightly in style and ordered so as to give an unbroken account of the case involved, but there are no changes in substance. In the original notes descriptions of the processing of more than one case were sometimes interspersed.

References

Elliot, Henry C. (1974), 'Similarities and Differences between Science and Commonsense', in Roy Turner (ed.), *Ethnomethodology* (Harmondsworth, Middx., Penguin).
Garfinkel, H. (1967), *Studies in Ethnomethodology* (Englewood Cliffs, New Jersey, Prentice-Hall).
Merrison Report (1975), *Report to the Committee of Inquiry into the Regulation of the Medical Profession* (London, HMSO).
Polanyi, Michael (1958), *Personal Knowledge: Towards a Post-critical Philosophy* (London, Routledge & Kegan Paul).
Roth, Julius (1974), 'Professionalism: The Sociologists' Decoy', *The Sociology of Work and Occupations*, Vol. 1, No. 1.
Roth, Julius and Douglas, Dorothy (1971), *The Utilization and Functioning of the Hospital Emergency Service*, Report to the National Institute of Health (Department of Sociology, University of California).
Sudnow, David (1967), *Passing On: The Social Organization of Dying* (Englewood Cliffs, New Jersey, Prentice Hall).

The following paper presents a study in the status of medical knowledge. Drawing upon anthropology for her theory and diabetes for her example, Posner argues that certain aspects of medical practice should be seen as based not on science, but on myth and belief. According to medical orthodoxy, diabetes can be unambiguously diagnosed and treated. Once located, a diabetic will be placed under a regime to control his or her blood sugar level by regulating the amount of insulin. Members of the lay public may assume that such management is based on scientific consensus; Posner, however, offers us an alternative interpretation. She puts forward evidence which suggests that there is little scientific justification for the medical action taken. Further, she offers examples which illustrate that doctors continue such a practice despite acknowledged disagreement about its value. Why do they do this? Posner underlines the symbolic importance attached to regulation of the blood sugar level, and the belief in this ritual of 'control' held jointly by practitioners and patients. Indeed, she argues, such belief is an important mechanism for sustaining the practitioners' faith maintained in the face of uncertainty about the condition.

Not only is the management of diabetes built upon the practices of traditional magic, but the factors which influence the diagnosis of the condition also appear to be arbitrarily derived. Within the medical profession, 'normality' of blood sugar level is socially defined. Nevertheless, the labelling and identification of diabetes has important consequences for the sufferer's subsequent career — affecting both their social life and their employment prospects.

The nature of medical knowledge is difficult to study, for belief in the overriding strength of scientific fact is strong (and one to which this paper implicitly subscribes). A variety of perspectives have been employed in the attempt. Elsewhere in this book, for example, Hughes examines the commonsense grounding of medical knowledge in hospital practice, a line of argument which ethnomethodologists have extended to the study of science. This paper takes a different theoretical position, one which in its own way, serves to look behind accepted medical practice and question the assumptions upon which such practice has been built.

M.R.

MAGICAL ELEMENTS IN ORTHODOX MEDICINE:
Diabetes as a Medical Thought System

Tina Posner

This paper will look at the diagnosis and treatment of diabetes as a medical system within the wider medical system of orthodox Western medicine. I will attempt to examine the thinking behind the practice, and to show why the treatment can be viewed partly as a magical ritual. My starting-points are the presuppositional, analogical and circular nature of much scientific thought, and the rationality, within limits, of magical thought (see Bibliography). Important theoretical considerations are Horton's argument that the crucial difference between traditional and scientific thinking is that the traditional thinker is unable even to imagine possible alternatives to his established theories; and the suggestions of writers such as Kuhn and Polanyi that scientific thinkers, though they may admit alternatives, may nonetheless have a protective attitude towards established theory. Such protectiveness recalls Evans-Pritchard's discussion of the 'secondary elaboration' of the Azande in the face of the failure of their magic.

In a paper on 'Medicine's Symbolic Reality' Arthur Kleinman (1973) wrote:

> Medical systems employ different explanatory models and idioms to make sense of disease and give meaning to the individual and social experiences of illness . . . A given medical system in its socio-cultural context does considerably more than name, classify, and respond to illness, however. In a real sense, it structures the experience of illness and, in part, creates the form the disease takes.

My research involves an analysis of diabetes as a medical system as a whole, and this paper represents only the beginnings of that analysis.

I wish to take a definition of magic provided by Raymond Firth and use it as a framework within which to illustrate what I am calling the magical elements in the treatment of diabetes, as I have seen it and heard it spoken about. The illustrations will be drawn from my observations in a diabetic outpatient clinic and from interviews with doctors I have observed.[1] Firth (1958) suggested that 'magic as

Magical Elements in Orthodox Medicine 143

commonly accepted' is 'a rite or verbal formula projecting man's desires into the external world on a theory of human control, to some practical end, but as far as we can see based on false premises'. I will talk about the theory of human control – the rationale of diabetic treatment – as it has been presented to me. I shall also discuss the treatment itself, viewed as a protective ritual.

The practical end of the treatment of diabetes is to eliminate the patient's symptoms; secondly, to normalise a biochemical parameter – the blood sugar level – defined as 'abnormal' in diabetics according to its distribution in the general population; and, finally, to prevent or retard the development of diabetic complications, which can include peripheral neuropathy – loss of feeling at the extremities, gangrene and possible amputation, death from coronary thrombosis or a stroke, vascular disease, renal failure, impotence and loss of sight resulting from cataract or retinopathy.

The basic premises of the theory of the medical control of diabetes are that it is right to reduce the raised blood sugar level to a level defined as 'normal', i.e. approximating the average in the general population, and to maintain it at such a level. Such a reduction, it is argued, serves to eliminate symptoms and prevent or retard complications. Control of diabetes – 'control' is a key word in diabetic terminology – can be theoretically achieved and maintained by treatment with a diet eliminating sugar and restricting carbohydrate intake, or with a diet and tablets, or with a diet and insulin injections, depending on the severity of the diabetes. Treatments will reduce a raised blood sugar level and relieve the patient of symptoms (such as excessive thirst and passing an increased volume of urine), associated with a high blood sugar level. The main rationale of treatment, however, is the prevention, or at least, retardation of complications, and treatment will be initiated even when the patient has no symptoms, or continued after the patient's symptoms have been relieved, in an attempt to keep the blood sugar at a level held to be normal and safe. In the usual way, treatment would be continued for the rest of the patient's life with the importance of 'good control' being constantly stressed.

The basic hypothesis that the diabetes can be controlled by attempting to normalise the blood sugar level with the treatment available is far from established, however. No direct correlation has been shown between the severity of the diabetes and the development of complications, or between the degree of 'control' and the development of complications. Patients with mild diabetes may develop severe complications. Patients who have apparently been 'well controlled' may also develop complications. It is generally admitted there is room for doubt. One doctor interviewed said: 'at the moment we haven't got any terribly good evidence that rigidly controlling diabetes will prevent complications'. Later in the interview he said 'the few studies that have been done on this problem *do* indicate that rigid control *does* prevent complications. The evidence is *not good*. But there is *some* evidence pointing that way. There is *no* evidence . . . that if you leave them out of control they get less complications.' Another doctor I interviewed, pressed to explain why so much importance was attached to 'good control' in spite of the room for doubts about its efficacy, replied:

> The simplest answer to this is that although evidence is not weighted heavily in favour of good control reducing complications we all *secretly feel* that this is in fact the case, that if you can control the patient's diabetes as well as possible it *should* retard the development of complications. We all *secretly believe* this and *hope* about it, but there's no outstanding evidence that it is true.
>
> There have been a number of papers that support this, but a number of papers that don't support it.

Later he said, 'We want to find out the truth. It's not available at the moment'.

The first doctor in answer to the same question about the reason for such an emphasis on 'good control' in view of the admitted doubts explained:

> I think the reason is that the one thing that we can demonstrate wrong in diabetes is that the blood sugar is raised. It may not be the major factor in diabetes; there may be other more important factors – Such as? I asked.
>
> Maybe blood fats, maybe other biochemical changes which haven't yet been defined, maybe the type of insulin which is produced is abnormal. There may be other things which we don't know about yet. But the one thing we do know about is that people who have diabetes, by definition, really, have a raised blood sugar level and therefore it would seem logical to reduce the blood sugar. Also we know that patients with diabetes get complications and therefore we would assume at first sight that if you lower the blood sugar they wouldn't get complications. This would

be the first aim. And when it became possible to treat diabetes
with insulin, for example, it was not unnatural that people
wanted to try and rigidly control the blood sugar. And I suppose
a lot of our thinking is an overhang from that.

Later this doctor said: 'Although we're not sure that we're doing
good, until we've proved — until the answer has come out, most people
think it's unethical not to control the diabetes rigidly.'

At a seminar on 'The Education of Diabetic Patients' which I
attended, it was admitted by several doctors that 'we could be wrong
regarding good control reducing complications'. One doctor added
'But at least I won't be doing the patient harm'. The second doctor
whom I observed and subsequently interviewed was more open when
I asked him about the side-effects of treatment. He said:

... if a diabetic's got symptoms, you're obliged to treat him so
that he loses the symptoms. The problem patient is the patient
who doesn't have symptoms, but has a metabolic abnormality
of some sort, and at the moment, for want of any better treatment, we try and correct the metabolic abnormality as much as
possible with treatment in the hope that it will retard the
development of complications and make his life better. Well it
may be that the treatment we give in some cases causes more
complications than it saves ... we're in a difficult situation. We're
vulnerable.

I had been asking him about the frequency of comas resulting from
low blood sugar (hypoglycaemia, a complication of taking insulin),
as compared with comas resulting from high blood sugar, i.e. untreated
diabetes or diabetes completely out of 'control'. He said that *hypo*-
glycaemic attacks were 'much more common. It's the commonest of
all the complications of diabetes.' 'In other words,' I said, 'it's
treatment-induced. It's iatrogenic illness.' 'Treatment induced,'
he replied, and quoted me a survey which had showed that in long-
term diabetes the most common complication had proved to be
hypoglycaemic attacks resulting from taking insulin.

A basic rationale of treatment, to reiterate, is that it will prevent
or retard the development of the serious complications of diabetes
yet we have here an admission that the most common
complication of diabetics on insulin is a result of treatment.
It appears to be very difficult to get the blood sugar level just

right by artificial means and often insulin treatment overdoes it, so that the patient has too low a blood sugar level rather than a level that is too high. A low blood sugar level affects mental capacity amongst other things.

Disadvantageous complications may also arise from the tablets prescribed in the treatment of diabetes, as one doctor put it to me, 'The bad effects are that we don't know really whether they [the tablets] stop you getting complications or whether they actually cause complications.' There is considerable controversy and no clear picture seems to have emerged from the findings of surveys. In the USA tablets are not normally prescribed now since a very large-scale survey seemed to show that the two main drugs being used increased the risk of cardiovascular death in patients treated with those drugs. In this country what evidence there is has not supported the American findings, and tablets are widely and regularly prescribed in preference to insulin injections, where there is a choice, on the assumption that patients would prefer to swallow tablets than inject themselves.[2]

In reply to my questioning the justification of treating a patient with no symptoms with tablets, when there is some controversy about the possible ill effects of the tablets, doctors admitted that sticking strictly to a diet might well reduce the blood sugar level sufficiently in such cases. Sometimes patients are treated only with a prescribed diet. I asked one doctor what percentage of patients could be 'well controlled' on diet alone. He replied: 'A much greater proportion than in fact are at the moment. So in fact, too many people are on tablets.' The reasons he gave for this situation were that the patients had not been given adequate dietary instruction; that it had not been emphasised to them how important diet is; and that the patients did not stick to the diet for one reason or another. Another doctor, in reply to my question about why there was comparatively little emphasis on diet in spite of its admitted importance and apparent efficacy and the possible ill effects of tablets, replied:

> I think for a number of reasons. Mainly doctors and patients feel that by giving tablets you're practising real medicine, or by giving insulin, and by putting someone on a diet you're not really practising real medicine . . . But there's lots of very good evidence that if you severely restrict the carbohydrate content of the diet you can control the diabetes in a large percentage of cases.

In the outpatient clinic which I observed, patients saw the dietician when they were first diagnosed as diabetic for a session of dietary instruction. A diet was worked out with the patient within the level of restricted carbohydrate intake set by the doctor, and they were told which foods were completely prohibited. Patients were given some explanation, advice and encouragement, but no follow-up appointments were made because there were insufficient staff to cope with them. They were told to come back to see the dietician if they had some dietary problem. The doctor could refer them back if he thought it necessary. I only saw one of the four doctors I watched refer old patients to the dietician on occasions. This doctor, a consultant, and well-known specialist in diabetes, had been the co-author of a report of a survey a few years earlier which had found that 31 per cent of the sixty patients, whose tablets were stopped for a time, did not need the tablets if they kept to a suitable diet. There is widespread agreement that diet is an all-important aspect of treatment, but disagreement about the best dietary policy and considerable differences in dietary practice between diabetic clinics. It is only relatively recently that dieticians have been seen as other than 'glorified cooks' (as the dietician in the hospital where I was observing put it to me). They are one of the 'professions supplementary to medicine' and they are nearly always female. It could be said that the present status of dieticians in the eyes of doctors and patients is not in accordance with the importance that diet has in *theory* in the treatment of diabetes. Besides, the substance, so to speak, of the diet is out of the doctor's control. As one doctor put it: 'Diet is something that the layman can get to grips with and it's a form of medication that he can manipulate himself and he's always got some theories about it, most of which are non-scientifically based.' A prescription of tablets or injections can be controlled far more accurately by the doctor alone. And medicine is about tablets and injections of course, not menus!

I shall now consider efforts made to protect the hypothesis that controlling the diabetes by attempting to normalise the blood sugar level will prevent or retard complications. This claim is made in the face of the lack of good evidence to support it and the evidence of complications arising from the treatment itself.

Firstly the medicine itself can be blamed. The pharmaceutical companies are constantly developing new tablets with modifications and claimed improvements on the older tablets, and attempting to develop more highly purified insulin which, it is hoped, will produce fewer antibodies. If the blood sugar is not at the desired level the most likely thing the doctor will do is to alter the prescribed tablets or insulin in some way — raising or lowering the dose or altering the type.

Secondly, the patient can be blamed. If he has not kept to the 'rules' how can he expect things to be all right? A patient who had collapsed as a result of a hypoglycaemic reaction was asked by the doctor, 'How many are you taking? — Ten? I asked you to reduce it to nine.' 'It's difficult to know how many he's taking, that's the trouble' the doctor said in a loud aside presumably directed to the nurse and myself. On another occasion — 'The only thing wrong with him is a low I.Q.' Even if the patient takes the tablets or insulin strictly according to prescription, it it highly unlikely that he will never, perhaps inadvertently, break his dietary taboos. Patients often blame themselves and supply dietary explanations for variations in their physiological state.

Then there are also the 'things we cannot control'. The mother of a boy being seen by the consultant asked: 'I wonder whether the ups and downs in the sugar are to do with his age?' The consultant replied: 'What you've got to understand is that there are three things we can control — the amount of insulin; the amount of food he eats; and the amount of exercise he gets. There are other things we can't control. We can never get it quite perfect.'

Another mother, a diabetic herself, was very worried by her son's collapse at school as a result of hypoglycaemic reactions, and said to the consultant: 'You know me doctor, I cheat and I'm not so strict with myself; but we're so strict with Billy, so according to us he should be perfect. We can't understand why, if we're doing everything right, things are going wrong.' The consultant replied that there were 'things over which we have no control' and changed the type of insulin.

Additional theories can be produced in support of the hypothesis. One doctor quoted earlier, said '... it may well be that the treatment we give in some cases causes more complications than it saves'; then, feeling understandably vulnerable, continued:

> But I could say one thing, that if one takes a somewhat technical example, if a patient has a blood sugar of 180, it means that his pancreatic beta cells are continuously being exposed to a blood sugar of 180 and therefore they are continuously being subjected to stress and continuously being forced to secrete insulin at a maximal rate. This will exhaust the beta cells and cause them to function poorly. Now if you can lower the blood sugar by any mechanism to 100 and keep it there, then there is less pressure on the beta cell, the beta cell will have to secrete less insulin and it will therefore

recover to some extent, and the recovery will be associated with an increased secretion of insulin and the patient therefore, once you've brought him down from 180 to 100, may well be able to keep himself down there. Now if you'd left him at 180 his beta cells might have got more and more tired and his sugar would have just gone up. Now it's a *theoretical* situation which I'm *sure* happens in *practice*. If you bring down the sugar and let the pancreas rest then its function will be improved. Since it's insulin deficiency which causes complications, it's *reasonable* to *suppose* that this is a good thing for the patient.

Blame can then be attributed to the inadequacy of the means of monitoring the patient's blood sugar level. The same doctor quoted above also said:

If we're looking at diabetic control we ought to think of all the biochemical variables such as lipids, proteins, lipoproteins — hundreds of things really and one really ought to measure the whole spectrum to see (a) whether they're normal at a point value in time and (b) whether they're normal throughout the day, and obviously you just can't do this. So really ideally diabetic control is when the diabetic's biochemical variables are the same as yours or mine, and we never ever achieve it, and this may well be why diabetics still get complications when their sugars seem to be apparently in the normal range.[3]

It was this doctor who had told me earlier that:

... if you make an experimental animal diabetic by taking away insulin from it by a pancreatectomy or giving it drugs, then that animal, even when maintained on insulin will develop all the complications of diabetes and will develop all the metabolic abnormalities of diabetes. So, in other words, by changing one aspect of the body's metabolism, merely taking the insulin molecule out of the system you cause a myriad of secondary problems and abnormalities.

This doctor however carried on treating diabetes, basing his assessment of the metabolic state of the patient, on a measure of blood sugar level alone.

Writing about diabetes, Cochrane (1972) makes the following points:

In general the treatment of mature diabetics would seem to be an example of the large-scale use of ineffective and possibly dangerous therapies in a particularly inefficient way. The cause of the sad situation seems to be the assumption that if some bio-chemical parameter is abnormally distributed in a defined group of people, 'normalizing' the distribution must do more good than harm. In mature diabetes it may well be the wrong parameter that is being altered.

In spite of medical awareness that other biochemical parameters are involved in this metabolic disorder which may be as, if not more, important, doctors feel they are 'very justified', indeed, that it would be 'unethical' not to attempt to normalise the blood sugar level which by definition is abnormal in diabetics. With the discovery of insulin, the blood sugar level could be lowered and to some extent, controlled. The whole specialism of diabetes grew up around this ability. Other relevant biochemical parameters are not at present under the doctor's control to anything like the same extent, although they can be measured. I asked one doctor if he would want other things to be measured at the same time as the blood sugar level, such as the blood lipids. He replied: 'No, I don't think so, not in the present state of knowledge. I think it's the only thing we can go by at the moment.'[4] It was the same doctor who also said '. . . the one thing that we can demonstrate wrong in diabetes is that the blood sugar is raised. It may not be the major factor in diabetes, there may be other more important factors. . .'

The blood sugar level and its regulation is, then, all important in the treatment of diabetes as it has evolved — treatment which can be viewed in part at least as a protective ritual to ward off the threat of complications arising.

I shall now examine parts of this ritual purporting to control the diabetes. The essential feature as far as the doctor is concerned, is the monitoring and regulation of the blood sugar level. At the diabetic clinic under observation, this level was measured from a blood test at each visit. One of the doctors interviewed, encouraged by my earlier questions, speculated:

I mean the whole business about diabetic clinics. Whether it's necessary to run a diabetic clinic in the way that we do, is open to doubt also. You know — what relevance does one blood sugar pay to the rest of the time?
You mean the blood sugar measured at 1.30 p.m. on a Wednesday

afternoon. Did you have some doubts about it?

He backtracked somewhat saying:

> I felt reassured by it. In general I'd say the blood sugar did seem to match up fairly well and probably more important is that most patients with diabetes, even, no matter what their I.Q. is, understand that a high level of blood sugar meant their diabetes is bad, and if they could actually see the figure, it's the thing they count on most.

The patients often said 'How is my diabetes', meaning what is my blood sugar. This doctor's emphasis on the *symbolic* importance of the blood sugar level measurement is significant.[5]

There is some recognition that the measurement of the blood sugar level at one point in time could well be unrepresentative, and that such a measurement could have drawbacks as a criterion of control of the diabetes. Another doctor told me:

> Unfortunately the blood sugar fluctuates a lot during the day and a lot from day to day and even more from week to week. So a point value of blood sugar is rather a dangerous thing to base a change of treatment on.
> ... I think it's slightly flimsy evidence of poor diabetic control. If a patient's got a very high sugar of about 480 and they're running ketones in their urine and 2% sugar, well obviously, they're not controlled properly. If a patient's got a blood sugar of 90 and their urine's clear then obviously they are controlled; but there's a host of things in between that could either mean poor or good diabetic control and this is a weakness in the system it's difficult to overcome.

Consideration of the medical construction of reality and claims to certainty (Maclean, 1974) are every relevant here, and in the examination of the main diagnostic test for diabetes. One of the doctors I observed spoke to a patient of a 'special test which will *prove one way or the other* whether you have got diabetes'. The test he was referring to was the glucose tolerance test — a four-hour test during which the body's response to a large dose of glucose (administered orally or intravenously) is plotted by testing the blood sugar level. It was admitted to me that 'the definition of an abnormal glucose tolerance curve is variable depending on which centre you work at'. An experiment on prison inmates where the experimenter could standardise the variable factors affecting the test to an extent impossible in normal circumstances, found that a large number of individuals were never diabetic, some were always diabetic, and some were sometimes diabetic and sometimes not, on routine criteria. Arthur Mirsky (1970), writing about the 'Certainties and Uncertainties in Diabetes Mellitis' suggested that:

> Too frequently little or no consideration is given to the fact that the variation between successive tests in the same subject may be as great as the variation between subjects; that a test may be apparently abnormal one day and normal thereafter. Likewise, the influence of age, sex, prior diet, prior medication, posture, emotional state, physical activity, and many other factors is frequently disregarded in evaluating the clinical significance of a conventionally defined abnormal tolerance curve. Since the tolerance for glucose, as judged by standard criteria, decreases with age, all of us will become 'chemical' diabetics if we live long enough.

Another medical writer (Schwartz, 1968) has emphasised: '... a mildly abnormal glucose tolerance curve does not establish the diagnosis of diabetes ... Nor does a normal test provide any real assurance that a patient is free of diabetes and its consequences.'

Mirsky questioned the *propriety* of making such designations as 'asymptomatic', 'subclinical' or 'chemical' diabetes, irrespective of the validity of the criteria used to evaluate the response to a glucose load, because such designations may initiate iatrogenous consequences. He would think it more valid to view a person's tendency to the metabolic disorder involved in diabetes in terms of the minimum and maximum limits of their particular physiologic system. He writes: 'The mere fact that one system has a capacity which is poor relative to others does not mean that that system is necessarily inadequate. Inadequacy can be described only as a result of the interaction between the system and the particular circumstance to which it succumbs.' (p. 994.) Classically diabetes is described as a clinical syndrome characterised by polyphagia, polydipsia, and polyuria, loss of weight and other signs and symptoms attributable to hyperglycaemia, glycosuria and other consequences of a disordered metabolism of carbohydrate fat and protein. Nowadays, relatively few patients come to the doctor with this overt syndrome. Often they come with a variety of complaints related to some vascular or neurological disorder, or without symptoms, and only as a result of a routine medical examination has sugar been found in the urine. If they are defined as diabetic according to the standard criteria they will be labelled and treated as 'diabetic'. This labelling may have an important bearing on the type of job which will be open to the patient thereafter. and, remember, it is assumed that once a diabetic always a diabetic — the label is permanent[6]; and if his tests were only marginally abnormal they might have been normal had he come at another time; and who sets the criteria on which the tests are based? I heard one doctor say: 'Diabetes is what I say it is.' It is openly admitted that the NHS could not cope with the number of diabetics who would be found on a large-scale screening programme.

It is important to point out that it may be very misleading to think of all the patients classified as diabetic according to the standard tests, as having the same metabolic disorder. 'Diabetes is undoubtedly a group of diseases', I was told by one doctor. There is a definite distinction to be made between 'juvenile-onset' diabetics (in which the ability of the pancreas to produce insulin is very limited or absent); here, patients need insulin and would die without it sooner or later with *hyper-* glycaemic coma and ketoacidosis; and 'mature-onset' diabetes which normally occurs in a much milder form and sometimes may be a transient consequence of obesity and corrected by a suitable diet, it seems. Mirsky (1970) concluded:

> The only consensus that can be reached from the evidence available at the present time is that diabetes mellitus in man is a complex of at least two related syndromes. One syndrome is characterized by signs and symptoms attributable to a decreased availability of insulin to the cells. The other is characterized by signs and symptoms of vascular damage attributable to an independent defect in the metabolism of the vessels. Either syndrome may precede the other, each may occur without the other, or both may occur together. It is quite possible, however, that one may aggravate the other. (p. 992.)

Mirsky also pointed out that vascular derangements occurred very frequently in diabetics and were regarded as complications of the metabolic disorder termed diabetes.[7] As we have seen, a basic rationale of treatment of the diabetes is that 'good control' will have a preventative effect on the development of such complications. Often, however, vascular derangements occur among diabetics whose diabetes has been 'well controlled' and the manifestations of such pathological changes may be fully evident before the diabetes produces any symptoms. Mirsky adds:

All efforts to establish a definitive direct causal relationship between the severity of the metabolic derangement and the various types of vascular degeneration have been unsuccessful.

Recognition that vascular derangements may be antecedents or concomitants rather than consequences of the metabolic derangement induces uncertainty where once there was certainty. (p. 992.)

How is it that the basic hypothesis we have been examining has not been seriously challenged and replaced? The definition of magic which we took at the beginning of this paper was 'a rite or verbal formula projecting man's desires into the external world on a theory of human control, to some practical end, but as far as we can see based on false premises' I have tried to show how the theory of the medical control of diabetes is based on unproven and, at the least, questionable premises. It has become evident that to some extent at least, acceptance of the basic hypothesis is a question of faith –

> ... we all secretly feel that this is in fact the case, ... we all secretly believe this and hope about it, but there is no outstanding evidence that it is true.

At the seminar mentioned earlier, the doctor initiating the discussion spoke provocatively of 'the confidence trick regarding good control reducing complications' which doctors perhaps perpetuated in an attempt to try to involve the diabetic 'into accepting or rejecting the philosophy'. There was general admission amongst the doctors that they could be wrong about the importance of 'good control' of the blood sugar level in the prevention of complications. But there was an overwhelming impression of confidence that they were not, and that the right thing to do was to treat as they had been doing, and that treatment would do more good than harm. 'The onus should be on the patient to ask questions' it was said. 'After all, the medical profession', said one doctor, 'is the only profession that one does automatically believe in.' Security indeed for a profession if it can claim the privilege of being presumed to know best, when members of it themselves admit that they do *not* know.

I now wish to suggest that the medical theory of the treatment of diabetes is a belief system which is sustained by certain medical assumptions and, like any other, by social, structural and cultural factors. The application of strictly scientific criteria to diagnosis and treatment would change the whole nature of the disease and the specialism which has grown up to treat it. Doctors involved in treating diabetes are faced with a situation of very great uncertainty. In many relevant areas they lack knowledge based on the firm foundations of statistically valid empirical research. Further uncertainty arises from the many factors beyond their control which effect the metabolic disorder defined as diabetes, and from the unpredictability of the onset of serious and life-threatening complications associated with the disorder. They have made it their job to treat a condition which they cannot cure and which may be degenerative. The need to feel that they can at least control it, and that there is something they can do which will help prevent complications is understandable. There is a predisposition to act rather than leave things alone and an assumption that the mistake of judging a sick person well is more to be avoided than judging a well person sick — a decision rule for handling situations of medical uncertainty described by Scheff (1963), who then suggested that the assumption on which this norm was based led to a situation where 'Physicians and public typically over value medical treatment relative to non treatment as a course of action in the face of uncertainty and this overvaluation results in the creation as well as the prevention of impairment.'

'The function of magic', Malinowski (1925) wrote, 'is to ritualize man's optimism.' Here we have doctors purporting to control diabetes, a metabolic disorder which they know involves a complex of biochemical parameters, through the manipulation of one such parameter over which they have incomplete control. Further, they insist that maintaining 'good control' of this parameter is essential to the prevention or at least retardation of complications associated with the disorder, when there is no good evidence to support this hypothesis. If they are not convinced they are doing the right thing, then they 'feel', 'believe', and 'hope' they are. They have faith in the efficacy of their ritual. Optimism is essential in the face of the unpredictability of the development of complications.

I should like to end by quoting from a book by Francis Hsu (1952) which discusses the measures taken to combat a cholera epidemic in a town in West China:

> ... if we follow the thoughts and ways of a culture as expressed through the bearers of the culture, magic and real knowledge are not only intertwined, but may not even be distinguished, so that, for reaching one and the same end, the individual oscillates between one and the other, or resorts to both simultaneously, with the greatest facility and ease of mind ... this lack of discrimination ...

is common to human behaviour in general ... man fails to differentiate between magic and science not because he lacks any power of rationality, but because his behaviour in general is dictated by faith developed out of the pattern of his culture.

Notes

1. These interviews were tape recorded. The observation was carried out in a large London teaching hospital. Notes were made of the doctor-patient interaction and parts of the conversation written down. Three doctors were observed. Since the time the paper was written further observation has been carried out in another outpatient clinic and three other doctors subsequently interviewed.
2. In a recent article in the *B.M.J.* (*B.M.J.*, 1976, 1, pp. 509-11) J. N. Stowers wrote: 'The bright prospects of tablet treatment have recently been marred by reports of increased cardiovascular mortality in patients taking the sulphonylurea tolbutamide, to be followed a little later by even worse results with the biguanide phenformin, compared with patients treated by diet alone or diet and insulin.

    'Evidence is by no means one sided but there seems to be little doubt that sulphonylurea drugs are associated with an increased mortality rate after myocardial infarction. Such considerations must temper our approach to the treatment of long term diabetes and more and better trials are needed to compare the cardiovascular risks of treatment with insulin and sulphonylureas.'

    (There are two types of tablet used in treating a raised blood sugar level, the sulphonylureas and the biguanides.)

    The article was entitled 'Modern Approach to Diabetes Mellitus-I' and was mostly a summary of tablet treatment and possible side-effects.

    Hypoglycaemia is a possible side-effect of tablet treatment too, particularly with certain sulphonylurea drugs with a long biological half-life. This type of hypoglycaemia is harder to treat than the transient type due to insulin overdose. The drug persists in the blood a long time and glucose needs to be given by continuous infusion over many hours and not just as a single intravenous dose as is the case after an overdose of short-acting insulin.

    There are other possible side-effects, such as rashes. 'The therapeutic dose of biguanides', Stowers wrote, 'is often near to the dose which will start to produce side-effects, which occur in the following order: anorexia, nausea, and then vomiting or diarrhoea, or both, with associated malaise.'
3. 'The effect of control on long term complications has not been established because we have no real measure of day-to-day control of the disease.' (Alex Wright, *Modern Medicine*, June 1976, pp. 30-4.)
4. It is known that diabetes is associated with a raised cholesterol level in the blood, which in turn has been shown to be associated with a rise in the mortality from ischaemic heart disease. Ischaemic heart disease is considered to be a possible complication of diabetes, and it is known that diabetics are prone to it. It is possible to lower the level of blood cholesterol by using a drug called Atromid S (Chlorophibrate).
5. In my observations and recordings in the outpatient clinic I have noted many instances of the patient's diabetes being treated as if equivalent to

his blood sugar level by both doctor and patient alike. Because of the importance of the symbolic meaning of the blood sugar level for the patients, there might be some difficulty in their accepting the measurement of other blood levels known to be significantly associated with a raised blood sugar level and any attempt to alter these by more drugs.

6. Although this is the assumption – a section in the 'Diabetics' Handbook' published by the British Diabetics Association, for instance, starts 'Diabetes is for life . . .' the medical profession recognises that in some cases of mature-onset diabetes the condition may be transient.
7. Vascular derangements are involved in most of the conditions considered complications of diabetes. 'About 20% of new diabetics presenting to clinics already have recognisable diabetic complications', according to Stowers in the *B.M.J.* article cited earlier.

References

1. Cochrane, A. L. (1972), *Effectiveness and Efficiency: Random Reflections on Health Services* (The Nuffield Provincial Hospitals Trust), pp. 56-7.
2. Firth, Raymond (1958), *Human Types*, revised edn. (New York, Merton Books), p. 124.
3. Hsu, Francis L. K. (1952), *Religion, Science and Human Crises* (London, Routledge & Kegan Paul), p. 8.
4. Kleinman, Arthur M. (1973), 'Medicine's Symbolic Reality. On a Central Problem in the Philosophy of Medicine', *Inquiry*, 16 (2), pp. 208-9.
5. MacLean, Una (1974), *Patient Delay: Some observations on medical claims to certainty* (Dept. of Community Medicine, Univ. of Edinburgh).
6. Malinowski, Bronislaw (1925), *Magic, Science and Religion and other Essays* (New York, Doubleday Anchor Books), p. 90.
7. Mirsky, I. Arthur (1970), 'Certainties and Uncertainties in Diabetes Mellitis', in Max Ellenburg and Harold Ritkin (eds.), *Diabetes Mellitis: Theory and Practice* (McGraw Hill, 1970).
8. Scheff, Thomas J. (1963), 'Decision Rules, Types of Error and their Consequences in Medical Diagnosis', *Behavioural Science*, 8.
9. Schwarz, T. B. (1968), 'Who is a diabetic?', *Ann. Intern. Med.*, 69, p. 161.

Bibliography

Armstrong, David, 'The Changing Basis of Medical Knowledge', Unit of Sociology, Guy's Hospital Medical School, Oct. 1975, unpublished paper.
Barnes, Barry, *Scientific Knowledge and Sociological Theory* (London, Routledge & Kegan Paul, 1974).
Barnes, S. B., 'Paradigms – scientific and social', *Man*, N. S., 4, 1969.
Beattie, J. M. M., 'On Understanding Ritual', in Bryan R. Wilson (ed.), *Rationality* (Oxford, Basil Blackwell, 1970).
Douglas, Mary, *Purity and Danger*, (London, Routledge & Kegan Paul, 1966).
——— *Natural Symbols* (London, Barrie and Rockcliffe, The Cresset Press, 1970).
——— (ed.), *Rules and Meanings* (Harmondsworth, Penguin Education, 1973).
Evans-Pritchard, E. E., *Witchcraft, Oracles and Magic Among the Azande* (London, Oxford Univ. Press, 1937).
Firth, Raymond, *Human Types* revised edn. (New York, Merton Press, 1958), chap. VI, 'Reason and Unreason in Human Belief'.
Hollis, Martin. 'The Limits of Irrationality' in *Rationality*, Bryan R. Wilson (ed.) (Oxford, Basil Blackwell, 1970).

——— 'Reason and Ritual', in Bryan R. Wilson (ed.), *Rationality* (Oxford, Basil Blackwell, 1970).
Horton, Robin, 'African Traditional Thought and Western Science', in Bryan R. Wilson (ed.), *Rationality* (Oxford, Basil Blackwell, 1970).
Horton, Ribin and Finnegan, Ruth (eds.), *Modes of Thought* (London, Faber & Faber, 1973).
Hsu, Francis L. K., *Religion, Science and Human Crises* (London, Routledge & Kegan Paul, 1952).
Jarvie, I. C., and Agassi, Joseph, 'The Problem of the Rationality of Magic', in Bryan R. Wilson (ed.), *Rationality* (Oxford, Basil Blackwell, 1970).
Kleinman, Arthur M., 'Medicine's Symbolic Reality. On a Central Problem in the Philosophy of Medicine'. *Inquiry* 16 (1973), pp. 208-9.
Kuhn, T. S., *The Structure of Scientific Revolutions*, 2nd edn (University of Chicago Press, 1970).
Lukes, Steven, 'Some Problems about Rationality' in Bryan R. Wilson (ed.) *Rationality* (Oxford, Basil Blackwell, 1970).
MacLean, Una, *Magical Medicine* (Harmondsworth, Penguin Books, 1971).
Malinowski, Bronislaw, *Magic Science and Religion and Other Essays* (New York, Doubleday Anchor Books, 1954).
Marwick, Max, *'Is Science a Form of Witchcraft'*, *New Scientist*, 5 September 1974.
Peel, J. D. Y., 'Understanding alien belief-systems', *'British Journal of Sociology* 20 (1969).
Polanyi, M., *Personal Knowledge* (University of Chicago Press, 1958).

Time as a dimension of social life has traditionally been neglected by British sociologists. We have yet to produce incisive theoretical analyses to match those of Gurvitch or Moore, or research of the quality of Roth's on the structuring of time among tuberculosis patients. This collaboration between Joel Richman, a sociologist, and W. O. Goldthorp, a gynaecologist, has produced one of the first serious pieces of research to address this topic. Their paper starts from the social interaction between gynaecologist and patient in clinic sessions and they examine the ways in which an orientation to time permeates these encounters. Time has significance for diagnoses, as the gynaecologist establishes a history and assesses the temporal rhythms of a woman's life in menstruation, pregnancy, intercourse or the menopause. Time has significance for the organisation of the encounter as the gynaecologist and the patient bid to control its flow and to open and close discussions, examinations, questions or instructions. Time has significance for the organisations within which the encounters are set, as gynaecologists have to work with one eye on operating lists, waiting lists and clinic lists, the queues of cases of differing degrees of clinical severity whose priority must be matched against the availability of staff and resources. These constraints have their own consequences in terms of the relative priority which can be afforded to the time of patients and professionals.

Richman and Goldthorp provide few answers, but that is not their purpose. What they do is to alert us to a range of interesting and neglected questions and to one possible way of addressing them. The significance of this paper may lie less in the details of its argument, than in its inspiration for others. If knowledge is advanced by investigators standing on the shoulders of their predecessors, then this paper offers an unusually broad pair of shoulders which deserve to support the work of many who will come after.

R. D.

WHEN WAS YOUR LAST PERIOD?
Temporal Aspects of Gynaecological Diagnosis*

Joel Richman and W. O. Goldthorp

> Women are victims in the gynaecologist's waiting room, as they are in their own homes and elsewhere, of the assumption that a woman's time is of no value. Certainly, as between the doctor's time and the women's there is no question that the doctor's time receives the preference.
>
> (Kaiser and Kaiser, 1974)

Introduction

Our aim here is to present an account of some of the cultural features of the diagnostic processes in the setting of a gynaecological outpatient clinic. There is, of course, a voluminous literature on doctor-patient relationships. Much of this work has been derived from the experience of general practice, often involving, directly and indirectly, some discussion of the sick role, in debate with Parsons. Other studies have concentrated on analysing specific 'problems': for example, the communication of information (Waitzkin and Stoeckle, 1972); the termination of patient-practitioner relationships (Hayes-Bautista, 1976); client preferences of professional behaviour (Ben-Sira, 1976) and so on. Many studies operate with an explicit model of the structural form of the doctor-patient relationship; whether it be Szasz and Hollender's (1956) classification of activity-passivity, guidance co-operation, and mutual participation: or, conflict/bargaining models (Katz, Gurevitch, Peled and Danet, 1969). We intend to examine certain facets of patient/consultant[1] exchanges, especially the temporal strands involved in such relationships, which make it necessary to avoid superimposing an all-embracing model to 'freeze' the proceedings. More specifically, we hope to show how, in the consultation, mutual concern about time, in its multifaceted guises, becomes a domain activity which operates as both a topic of enquiry and a resource for developing explanations to achieve a provisional resolution of the often conflicting demands and beliefs of

---

* We are grateful to John Phillips, Jim Lord and Boris Allen for their lively and much appreciated critical comments on the paper. We also had the benefit of reading Sally Macintyre's then unpublished paper, 'To Have or To Have Not: Promotion and Prevention of Childbirth in Gynaecological Work'. Not least, many thanks are due to Elizabeth A. Nelles for typing the paper.

patient and gynaecologist. In so doing, we shall highlight some of the dilemmas, moral and technical, of the gynaecologist. As members of an occupational group, with its own identity, practices and beliefs they have to manage an outpatient list within an organisational context of increasing temporal turbulence. Both internally and externally others are increasingly circumscribing the limits of the gynaecologist's activities.

The temporal dimension, as an organising framework of analysis, has been singled out for a number of reasons. One common feature of doctor talk about the clinic is of how they are 'constantly fighting time'. The common element of both patient's and gynaecologist's practical reasoning centres on temporal consideration. Medicine throbs continuously with the taking of patient's histories: junior doctors are reminded incessantly by their mentors that 'good' histories are essential for successful diagnosis and treatment. The medical theories used by doctors assume that patients are sensitised to, and critically record, the passage of time as an everyday process — an essential prerequisite for self-medication, the most important ingredient of treatment regimes. The gynaecological consultation, like others, can be conceptualised as a mechanism for rewriting, in a formal and sometimes legal way, a patient's past and pointing out guidelines for future events. Not least, gynaecology is a unique specialism in its longitudinal investment in women from pediatrics to geriatrics.

Other studies of gynaecological encounters have not focused directly on temporal themes. From the USA, both Emerson (1970) and Henslin and Biggs (1971) have made the central theme of their analysis the problems involved in managing the setting for carrying out the necessary vaginal examination (V.E.). Both distinguish techniques for neutralising the multiple disruptive tendencies of the sexual connotations. Henslin's study is clearly an example of private medicine in a general practice, although he does not think it worthy of comment. Emerson's study (p. 88) introduces more patient typifications: the 'intractable' patient, the 'Southern Belle', the 'young' and the 'unmarried'. However, many crucial social parameters of the gynaecological examination receive scant attention and both papers are directed towards the construction of the generalised patient. The relevance of the temporal dimension is never made explicit. We are not told of the gynaecologist's orientations towards his work, the ordering of his priorities according to available resources and his position within the medical networks. Macintyre's study (1976) largely rectifies these omissions. However, her analysis is narrowly slanted towards one gynaecological face: the reconciliation of the paradox between the pro- and anti-natalistic aspects of their work. Because this has been covered in depth, we have, justifiably, not discussed patient's requests for terminations and sterilisations.

Any study is forced to foreclose and declare its 'limits of naivety' (Gluckman, 1964), beyond which it loses its momentum. Accordingly, we are aware of the current debates on the demands for a new 'social gynaecology', but it is not intended here to organise the analysis so as to present 'evidence' for or against such advocacy.

A Comment on the Methodology of Investigation

The main mode of presentation will follow that now distinguished as the ethnography of speaking, with its emphasis on what Bauman and Sherzer (1974) have called 'performance'; a way of speaking, which involves more than an etic list of communicative means, like codes. Briefly, the view is taken that knowledge of the rules of grammar is inadequate, *per se*, for understanding speech, meanings, and social transactions. Speaking is meshed in the cultural forms of settings and institutions where members bring their competencies, strategies, views, expectations and goals. The 'nexus of all these factors is performance', argue Bauman and Sherzer and they characterize it with 'emergent' properties, i.e. although it is possible to recognise and construct a 'standard' description of a patient-gynaecological consultation, every performance contains the potentiality for developing its own uniqueness. Some do become unique, depending on the communicative mix, individual competencies and goals, etc. For example, when juniors are present performances can deviate radically: they last longer; procedures and packages of questions asked of patients are duplicated; there are more pronounced breaks between medical talk and everyday talk. Similarly, one of our purposes will be to show how patients can emerge as 'special', as the consultation progresses and produce different concerns with time.

The choice of the ethnography of speaking as a vehicle for portraying the consultation was deliberate. When a medical specialist and sociologist are co-researchers it is important for them to find a common research technique that is fluid, mutually intelligible and penetrates both disciplines.[2] Ethnography demands extensive details of settings, to which the sociologist is an outsider and must remain so. To this end the medical specialists' knowledge is invaluable; they are performers, interpreters and informants. Furthermore, gynaecologists recognise the consultation as a 'verbal art form' (Bauman, 1975). One interpretation of their role is that of storyteller; their narratives contain stylistic responses; their audience is not only the immediate setting of the consultation, but can also be, simultaneously, the wider community they know to operate 'out-there'. Medicine has long been rooted in an oral tradition.[3] Consultants' speech acts are the major source of their authority for achieving 'successful' outcomes in the clinic. Women, too, attempt to tell stories, of their misfortunes.

The Gynaecological Consultation

The proceedings here cannot be fully understood without first noting the 'frontiers of control' screening the consultation and which assist the gynaecologist to produce 'predictable' outcomes. Two important factors can be mentioned: the composition of the clinic[4] list and the woman's prior knowledge of biological and medical explanations. The list is deliberately constructed with a blend of patients whose initial signs point towards known and usual allocations of time in consultation. Infertility cases, for example, need extensive use of talk. These women are usually very anxious. Women whose planned stay on the pill has been completed expect to conceive immediately. The range of information requested in a first interview can be extensive — covering such matters as the heat conditions at a husband's place of work, as well as those about coital behaviour. These consultations are unusual, for medical and biological terminology are frequently used. The gynaecologist directly attempts to educate the infertile woman (couple) to monitor accurately for him the fluctuations of body temperature and other temporal cycles. Over time the patient/gynaecologist relationship can resemble a 'quasi-colleagueship' one. She can become 'special' and be taken out of the formalistic sequencing of an outpatient list. Patients indicating post-menopause bleeding are initially categorised as potential cancer cases. The menstrual history has to be carefully scrutinised to distinguish from the patient's account between a 'heavy' period that is 'normal' from 'intermittent' periods which are not and, from a medical perspective, really means continuous bleeding. Cases indicating vaginal discharges and prolapses are more routine and require less time.

The patient's ignorance of her anatomy facilitates the gynaecologist's sequencing techniques. Our recent study of 250 hospitalised gynaecological patients (Goldthorp, Richman, 1974a) showed only two-thirds could give a 'recognisable' reason for their admission. The illness label recalled by many was emblematic rather than showing a 'deep' understanding of their condition. Over one-third did not know which organs had been treated/removed. Their body percept resembled that described by Manning and Fabrega (1973, p. 266) for the Chiapas Indians of Mexico in which the 'body can be described as an unrefined, undifferentiated, and largely unarticulated "black box" '. One common error was to regard the medical and lay term for the same organ as being two distinct parts, e.g. the uterus and womb and cervix and the neck of the womb were not considered the same organs. The constant truncating of the consultation by the gynaecologist with everyday talk to the patient and medical talk to the nurse (or other medical personnel) reinforces this tendency.

One useful metaphor to deploy initially in overviewing the consultation is that of the 'liminal' stage of a *rites de passage*. Turner (1975, p. 252) has argued that 'liminality represents a levelling and stripping of structural status . . . an enhanced stress on nature at the expense of culture'. Accordingly, patients are submerged into new and general status categories, possessing the qualities, e.g. of fibroids, vaginal discharge or atypical smears. Although the patient/gynaecologist relationship is clearly an asymmetrical one it remains, nevertheless, an integral part of the occupational ideology that the 'consent' of the patient is paramount for successful outcomes. It is seen as a joint venture. To what the patient 'consents', must, of course, be within an ambit influenced by length of waiting lists, allocation of theatre times, hospital disputes, competence of junior staff and, not least, the gynaecologist's own immediate medical interests. The ordering of these factors is not fixed. The government policy to introduce itemised payments for birth control techniques has meant, for example, a dramatic increase in the number of coil insertions carried out in some units.

In practice the consultation is not one of 'spontaneous' continuity. It is heavily compartmentalised (irrespective of its overall duration), each segment hinged with appropriate speech behaviour. The patient is expected to maintain a respectful silence at the opening whilst the case notes are being read and before the close when the gynaecologist writes up. After offering an account of her troubles, the proceedings are suspended for the V.E. Gynaecologists introduce this topic with talk represented by verbal formulae, emphasising it as a mechanical event. The prognosis at the end is conveyed by ceremonial talk. The findings are portrayed as the natural consequences of the joint patient/ gynaecologist endeavours, and in that they tend to symbolise the unity and even 'sacredness' of the occasion. There are many other speech features. For much of the proceedings the nurse is the silent partner, rarely initiating an exchange. When the nurse addresses the patient, it is inevitably an occasion when the gynaecologist has problems. The usual speech pattern is for her to repeat, or rephrase, the gynaecologist's comments, and forge a link with the patient through which he will send his messages: 'Nurse tell her to push down one more time.' Even when no link is forged the nurse will cocoon the patient and use 'just talk'. 'Just talk' is offered as a speech convention with much of the significance Reisman (1974) has attributed to what he has identified as 'making noise' in Antigua. Analogously he relates noise to contrapuntalism found in music. During a painful V.E. a patient may loudly utter unlinked words, which will not be treated as speech expressions with rules for openings, nor just left to exist. With 'just talk' the nurse has a routine of offering praise, breathing deeply, and indicating a fabricated time scale of the almost completed task of the gynaecologist, irrespective of what the patient is 'saying'. So residual are some of the verbal sequences in the consultation that gynaecologists will activate them irrespective of whether the patient can understand English.

Now we go on to select some extracts from patient/gynaecologist talk to elaborate some of the underlying rules. The following illustrates a familiar exchange in a 'routine' case with a new patient towards the end of a list.

    Gyn.: Is it Mrs X?
    P.: Yes.
    Gyn.: Something coming down in P.V. [reads to self from notes.]
       Twenty-eight and four children?
    P.: Three.
    Gyn.: Three and one miscarriage?
    P.: Yes.
    Gyn.: You are quite fit and well apart from this lump?
    P.: Yes.
    [External Examination.]
    Gyn.: Put your feet together and let your knees flop apart.
    [Internal Examination.]
    Gyn.: Has this been getting bigger at all?
    P.: Yes, it's got slightly bigger.
    Gyn.: Oh, you've got a coil in as well?
    P.: Yes.
    Gyn.: Force down. Again . . . Again. Mmh. It's just there, isn't it?
    P.: Mmh.
    Gyn.: Okay. Pop your legs down. It's not a very bad prolapse that.
       [Gynaecologist commences his findings.]
    P.: No.

Gyn.: It's just that the back wall of the vagina is bulging down a bit.
P.: Mmh.

The Gynaecologist goes on to elaborate the findings, states the type of operation which could be done, the consequences of leaving it as it is; and warns of the danger of scarring, which could be present after an operation and its possible effects on intercourse. The first questions causing the patient to acknowledge the special identity transfixed to age and obstetric history contributes towards the legitimisation of her location in the gynaecological setting. She does not own her obstetric history and is forced to recognise a miscarriage as now being significant. Furthermore, the gynaecologist's questions are so designed as to produce verbal 'striations' which elicit and 'groove' 'Yes' and its equivalent tokens of agreement from the patient. The clustering of agreement responses has a number of effects. They help to promote the aura of consensus between the gynaecologist and patient. Once grooved into giving a 'yes sequence' it is difficult in everyday conversation to radically divert to a new topic of tangentially opposed substance. It is more difficult for the supine patient with little kinesic amplification to initiate disagreement. The word most frequently used by all gynaecological patients is 'yes' and its equivalents – a useful indicator of overall patient acquiescence. Surprisingly, this usage had not been noticed until it was brought directly to the attention of the participating gynaecologist.

This extract also illustrates other regular features. In a dispute, as here, over gynaecological/obstetric history it is paramount for the gynaecologist that his version becomes unassailable as soon as possible. This is the major springboard for launching his theories of causation of the patient's troubles and justifications for what is to be done next. If the patient's history is left doubtful then the gynaecologist's explanations lack a degree of validation. Thus, the gynaecologist forces the patient to recognise four major 'foetal interludes' not only for the sake of medical accuracy, but also in case he has to offer the patient an explanation of *her* prolapse, i.e. she has had an 'above average' number of pregnancies in a short period of time. The immediate confrontation with her symptoms, after she has identified herself, both from the GP's note and the information she gave earlier to the junior doctor, forces her to make a commitment to them from which it is not easy to depart. If the patient is put in a position of being able to self-define her troubles the gynaecologist may not only be in danger of losing control of her temporal sequencing of the session, but also can be faced with the possibility of having to provide explanations and opinions about other branches of medicine whose interests also interlock with gynaecology, like psychiatry and general surgery. Patients quite often try to use the gynaecologist's expertise to check out the competency of their GP and his treatment. Greetings like 'Good day'; 'How are you?' which could provide wide openings for the patient to initiate the information exchange are reserved for 'special' patients such as those known beforehand that will be difficult to examine, like bewildered octogenarians. These greetings are normal in the antenatal setting, partly because of the continuing relationships; but most women still do not interpret them as an 'invitation' for a long discourse: there are other limiting factors. (Gynaecologists comment on this lack of an opening greeting by arguing that the patient has already been 'greeted' by the junior who earlier took the history and that they are merely following through the same processes).

Symptom circumscribing techniques are dominant in the opening sequences of a consultation, but can be operated at any given stage. In the matching exchange the patient is encouraged to commit herself to a condition of general overall well-being: 'You are quite fit and well *apart* from this *lump*.' The gynaecologist is using the descriptor 'lump' in this context indicating the triviality of the troubles. With cancer patients the word has a different connotation and is rarely indexed in the same manner. Patients are frequently asked to approve the notion of 'well-being' being conceptualised as having definable and objective qualities which are a matter of simple arithmetical logic of plus or minus. It then legitimates the gynaecologist advocating and then pursuing the 'appropriate' course of action.

Patients may offer a cluster of symptoms; some of long occurrence, some immediate; some restricted to the pelvic area like vaginal discharges; some more generalised like 'dizziness'. To produce a natural theory of causation explicating these linkages, making them intelligible, and presenting them as a gestalt to the patient is regarded as beyond the competence of the gynaecologist in the time available. When patients have ramified gynaecological histories, often enacted at different hospitals, the gynaecologist attempts to telescope the episodes into a manageable central focus, and in the form of a unitary model. It is often the way that the temporality of such a theory gravitates to the woman's periods with their transcendent properties. The gynaecologist in this example has not met the patient before and is disadvantaged by not being able to claim a first-hand familiarity with and involvement in the past episodes of her history. Therefore explanations he may offer about the 'distant' past's interaction with the present symptoms are open to challenge by the patient.

> Gyn.: This is an entirely *new* thing. So the *main* thing is that your *periods* are *irregular.*
> P.: While I have always been a little bit irregular.
> Gyn.: [slowly] You mean right from ...
> P.: When I was little. I never ...
> Gyn. [fast] : Right from the word start when you were little. Yes.
> P.: The only time I was regular was when I was on the pill.
> Gyn.: Oh haah ... Mm.
> P.: I came off the pill because they were affecting my breasts.
> Gyn.: I see. So for how long have you been off the pill altogether now?
> P.: Mmm ... roughly about eight months.
> Gyn.: Nearly eight months. Yes.

Once the gynaecologist can construct a temporal model synchronising the emergent and now 'dominant' symptom of the period variations with its agreed patterning, then the more presentable will be the explanation offered to the patient. In many cases of 'irregular' periods the gynaecologist himself does not know the 'precise' medical reason, nevertheless an account is constructed for the patient on this mutually acknowledged feature. The often prescribed D and C (dilation and curretage — the 'scrape') has much the same medical, curative status as ECT has in psychiatry. It is thought to stimulate a new hormonal balance. (The D & C differs, of course, from ECT treatment in that it is also a diagnostic tool.) The widespread use and multiplicity of contraceptive pills, with their well-established lore, as well as being an additional complicating factor in diagnoses, also enables the gynaecologist to provide the patient with the malleable bases of readily acceptable explanations of the source of her troubles. The evidence becomes 'obvious' and is as logically premised 'all round her' as that rooted in the Azande witchcraft beliefs. In line 8, the patient is given a clear opening to resonate the details of the effect of the pill on her. The extract illustrates, too, how the gynaecologist will sometimes allow the patient to complete the meaning of his aborted utterance (line 4). This is an additional strategy for creating the tenor of mutual agreement by facilitating the picture that things are being worked out together. Another instance of the expression of common sentiments is in the final summing up when the gynaecologist often employs the collective 'we' in the proposed course of action: 'Now what I am thinking, *we* can send you to the Southern for some X-rays, as an outpatient, and that will stop your periods for good. *We* just bring forward by a month, or a year, something which is going to happen in any case.'

Another way the gynaecologist can use to reach a speedy agreement, is to open the consultation by offering what appears to be (and can often be) the total range of logical possibilities for an occurrence. Together with the patient evidence will be sought to justify the problem falling within the orbit of one of the predetermined explanations. A given remedial course of action then becomes obvious, automatic and necessary, as in this exchange.

> Gyn: What it boils down to is that you have had the coil fitted by the FPA. Is that right?
> P.: Yes.
> Gyn.: And you wished for it to be removed, they couldn't find it.
> P.: Yes.
> Gyn.: In other words it looks, eh . . . well it's one of two things that's happened. Either your tag has come off, or the thing has come out. It's one of two things isn't it?
> P.: Yes.

The gynaecologist often has difficulties in deciphering whether a patient's opening description of a symptom, especially of repetitive bodily function of a period, or urinating, as opposed to something 'new' and 'different', can be classified as medically abnormal. The patterning of the activities can be differentially associated with, for example, aging and can still be normal clinically. 'Lengthy' periods, 'irregular' periods, 'painful' periods, 'heavy' periods, 'short' periods, 'missed' periods can, in given contexts, be regarded as medically appropriate. This type of exchange shows how the gynaecologist, by rotating the occurrence of 'wetness' rapidly through 'stills' of common everyday practices, is able to normalise what was offered to him as a new and primary symptom. The patient is a former one who had a hysterectomy recently and was seeing the gynaecologist ostensibly about a new vaginal discharge. The 'stills' flashed before the patient of when 'wetness' can occur are both context free and atemporal. This prevents the patient from elaborating in depth the social significance of the occasions and contains the symptom within the defined bounds of medical time.

Gyn.: It's still a bit red isn't it?
P.: Yes it's a bit sore. I've had a leak, you know. A leak you know.
Gyn.: Where from?
P.: From the side.
Gyn.: If you sat down, or if you cough or sneeze?
P.: When I stand up.
Gyn.: When you stand up.
P.: Yes.
Gyn.: But if you have got to do something after it, what happens?
P.: If I've got to go to the toilet?
Gyn.: Yes.
P.: I've got to rush sometimes, you know.
Gyn.: I see.
P.: But during the day I am feeling a bit wet you know.
Gyn.: But nothing happens when you cough or sneeze?
P.: No.
Gyn.: Or laugh?
P.: No.
Gyn.: Or bend down or *stand up*?
P.: No, nothing.

By introducing the signs of discomfort from the past operation the patient accepted it as legitimate to enlarge the temporal horizon of medical relevance and diversify the range of symptoms. The 'interrogative' style of the exchange now adds constraint to the proceedings and nullifies the patient's original pronouncement that 'standing up' is the only occasion when she dribbles. The woman's original pronouncement didn't make sense to the gynaecologist; for 'strenuous' activities should also have made her dribble. The gynaecologist also possessed the counter-evidence of the physical examination. The patient's chronological age as well as its manifestations in obstetrics/gynaecological history now becomes the gynaecologist's supreme resource in presenting his explanation. Women in this category, hovering around the menopause, are often forced to acknowledge their age prior to the summing up. In the continuing dialogue the woman's original 'soreness' has been reclassified as 'reasonably well-healed'.

Gyn.: How old are you now? Fifty?
P.: Fifty-four. Fifty-five. [Softly.]
Gyn.: Well, fifty-four. You are reasonably well healed up at the

top, but what you have are post-menopausal signs there . . .
We have got the change of age in the front passage. And again
it tends to get thin and infected.

The gynaecologist's confrontation with patients over their age could be interpreted as an assault on one of the key props in their definitions of feminity. The speaker's device used by the gynaecologist to manipulate the above sequence for his own ends has been called by Churchill (1966) an 'invitation to balance'. It was not a total assault on the patient's self-definition. The gynaecologist did not initially use an all-embracing precise number, for the patient's chronological age as available to him from the records at hand. He also accepted the lower of the two ages offered by the patient. However, in other contexts it can be the patient who first tenders the information on age so as to force special recognition from the gynaecologist. An occurrence of this is when requests for sterilisation and terminations are made.

The gynaecologist can not only menace patients' self-definitions of their feminity/sexuality by ritually recalibrating them around their chronological age, but also undermining the lay theories they hold of the 'genesis' of their complaints. In making sense of their 'newly developed' backache, or inflammation, patients can often locate the onset with a now significant social event from the past. The account of the causation of their troubles is likely to have been sanctified, at least in part, by its repeated acceptance when tested in the company of others. For some, an integral expectation from the consultation is to receive the final 'benediction'[5] for their lay theory. In mundane cases, to accept, or incorporate, such an analysis into his medical scheme would mean that the patient could now rightfully claim a hand in steering the future course of events and shatter the gynaecologist's fragile time-tabling. Such topics as 'falls', 'parties', 'toilets' and 'other doctors' practices' figure prominently in the lay accounts of misfortunes. Another reason for the reluctance of gynaecologists to validate a patient's lay theory is because they do not know to what use it may be put outside the hospital. The woman controls the information and relays it between home and the hospital. A 'fall' in a story told to a gynaecologist could really be an assault by the husband. There are occasions when the gynaecologist and patient conspire to conceal information from the husband. Stimson and Webb's (1975) analysis of how women tell medical histories to their selected audiences is relevant here. Their study concerned the consultation in general practice and the GP was the central focus of these accounts. They argue that the rehearsal of these stories is a dramatic reaffirmation of the moral conduct to be expected ideally from their GP. The teller frequently appears in the stories as having more expertise than the GP in predicting the rightful outcome. The stories also provide guidelines for others as to how they should present themselves to doctors and evaluate their decisions.

In this example the summing up stage was reached and the gynaecologist was reassuring the patient that her bleeding was medically trivial and of general occurrence.

> Gyn.: It's just what we call cervicitis, you know. It's just uncomfortable, I know.
> P.: Well. [Cut off.]
> Gyn.: It certainly looks all there is to the naked eye.
> P.: A good while ago doctor . . .
> Gyn.: Yes.
> P.: I was washing my hair and children in the bathroom you know. . .
> Gyn.: Yep.
> P.: . . . and my foot was soapy and it slipped . . .
> Gyn.: Yep.
> P.: . . .and I banged myself, you know, and I bled a little bit after. I injured myself there. [Points to her back which had not been examined.] I thought it might have been the shock of falling you know.
> Gyn.: No. You may have sort of, er, *shaken* yourself. Even if it turns out that the smear test shows atypical cells. Right.
> P.: Yes.
> Gyn.: As opposed to normal cells it could be microscopic and would be a hundred per cent treatable.

When faced with the injection of a patient's new account at the *end* of a consultation, like this one, which is an invitation to restart the diagnosis anew, it becomes doubly unacceptable. It is noteworthy how even at the part of the consultation most restrictive to patient's interventions, the woman gains access to the dialogue by the use of the title 'doctor' which evokes the moral obligation of an acknowledgement. The immediate switch of topic by the gynaecologist to the problematics of cancer now transforms the case into a potentially serious one, and it is intended to subsume the special significance the patient accredits to her explanation of the same phenomenon.

Becoming Special

We want to introduce, briefly, the concept of the 'special patient'. Sudnow (1967, p. 171) has used the term 'special cases' when referring to those patients deemed by doctors to be either 'particularly obnoxious' or 'particularly worthy'. These extreme moral evaluations are constructed primarily from appearances and determine one's life chances on admission. The preconstituted type of being 'special' pertains to those patients, in gynaecological diagnosis, to whom the boundary of what is usually considered (for 'routine' cases) strictly medically relevant information, is no longer fixed. As the frontier extends to embrace more data of the social texturing of the complaint, then the patient's concepts of temporal ordering become more a prominent feature in the consultation. There are many subdivisions of being 'special'. Some patients are recognisable as being special before the consultation commences; others become special during the progress of the consultation. The first group consists of, for example, former patients, repeat patients undergoing treatments, 'professional' patients from other medical specialisms and new patients whose status one wishes to acknowledge because of their connections with medicine, the hospital, or the local community. The categories of 'special' and 'routine' patients does not match, in many cases, the categories of 'serious' and 'non-serious' illness categories. It does not follow, too, that 'special' patients are 'better' diagnosed, even though they may have been allowed to talk longer. A woman having cancerous tissue in the uterus can be 'routine' and have the same diagnosis as if she was 'special'. Diagnosis can be a continuous process and one not confined to the patient/doctor consultation. Extra information is always being fed to the gynaecologist from relatives, friends, social workers, other medics and, of course, there can be new evidence revealed during an operation. The circulation of patients who are 'special', because of their prior connections with medicine, has important consequences for the gynaecologist's other relationships. There are established etiquettes for this form of clientship involving all grades, within and between hospitals. Within the same department a nurse, technician or administrator may approach the gynaecologist directly about a relative's condition, if known personally by him. A nurse, or auxiliary, from another department will often ask the ward sister to approach the gynaecological sister, who then will approach the gynaecologist on their behalf. The circulation of some 'special' patients is analogous to the movement of Rossel Island currency (Baric, 1963). It can counterbalance the fissiparous tendency of competing medical units with symbolic ties of co-operation. Within one's unit favours extended to those at the lowest levels of the hierarchy helps to improve morale. Above all, the circulation of 'special' patients leads to a re-allocation of resources, over and above that determined by the economic logic of hospital budgets. Departments can develop interest, for example, in types of research not recognised by resource allocation and a 'special' patient from a department so favoured can lead to a pooling agreement between the two departments.

In the opening sequence of the consultation the identities of 'special' patients are immediately acclaimed. Repeat patients, or former patients, are often greeted with temporal markers, e.g. 'Well, it's two years since I last saw you', or 'Tell me what's been bothering you in the meantime.' They can often tell their story in their own way. The gynaecologist has on record from the previous meetings their essential medical profile, that now has the credentials of being residual fact. The onus for new elaborations is put on the patient and this is very much matrixed in social time. 'Professional' patients can have circulated widely through a number of medical branches, perhaps being referred originally from gynaecology and returning via psychiatry. The gynaecologist is forewarned by their voluminous case notes written in different medical styles. Their complex story has undergone many rehearsals and authenticity is built into it by the way they sprinkle specialists' names and lists of medical terminology for treatment regimes. Experience has shown that if these patienst are cut off abruptly when recounting their history, one forfeits their co-operation and the situation can rarely be restored unless the gynaecologist 'works hard' to make amends. The records from other specialists can be open to a number of gynaecological reinterpretations. Medical records never indicate what the patient was told at the time by the doctor in charge of the case. Clues from the patient, especially about the drugs administered to her, are essential. In fact her present gynaecological troubles may be due to the past drug regime. Another type of 'professional' patient is the woman who has passed her medical career in only one specialism, but that for a major complaint. The opening greeting here is one of sympathetic rapport, acknowledging her medical trajectory. 'They have been knocking you about a bit haven't they Mrs Jones? Mitralvalvectomy. So you have got one of those plastic affairs.' There is a tendency for gynaecologists to use the consultation to transform the patient into an object of medical curiosity and appreciate the latest techniques of another medical specialism — in this case heart surgery. These patients are usually deferential and very apologetic to doctors who are regarded as their 'saviours'. 'No, no, no, Mrs Jones you are not a nuisance. I'm going to get my stethoscope and I'm going to listen to those funny sounds you have in your chest.'

Patients can become 'special' as the consultation proceeds. Their differentiating quality could be that they have come tagged, in some way, with information the gynaecologist finds useful and which may not be strictly relevant to the medical task at hand. Patients are directed to the consultant by their GP. The process of activation within the GP referral network provides the gynaecologist with his first indication of the patient's condition. Some GPs' comments on patients are more trustworthy than others. Some GPs are known personally from their work in the hospital, as in the short-stay maternity section (GP Unit). Many GPs' notes merely say, 'Please see Mrs X and advise.' Another GP stipulates all his referrals are urgent cases and so on. During the consultation the gynaecologist is able to evaluate the changing pattern of the GP network. If he discovers a patient has come from a GP newly arrived in the area, the gynaecologist will widen the temporal characteristics of the diagnosis to prompt the patient into commenting on her new practitioner.

In general, the style of diagnosis with special patients, to use a crude dichotomy, is one of being 'patient-centred', as opposed to being 'symptom-centred'. With special patients the tendency is to demystify the proceedings and reduce the relevance of the hospital *rites de passage*. The effect is to inject into the setting the wider contexts of the patient's self with its multiple realities of temporal significance. The gynaecologist offers more words of praise and encouragement after patients comply with their instructions − 'Good, that's fine.' Instructions are cloaked as personal favours. With some patients there is joking relationship, with others, like ex-cancer patients, the relationship resembles a 'quasi-courtship' (Scheflen, 1965). Gynaecologists refer to some of the special patients as 'friends' − a category usually reserved for private patients. At the end of the V.E. when the findings are presented, he will personally assist the patient to sit up on the couch. This is the normal practice in the antenatal clinic. The patient-centred style of diagnosis produces problems for the gynaecologist. He can have great difficulty disengaging himself and making an exit. Not all patients approve of the style and regard some of the comments as irrelevant. Those who have invested a great deal of the self in the sick role regard the line of questioning as detracting from the major symptom issue. It is apparent that the patient-centred style − the epitome of the bedside manner eulogised in medical tests − is often inappropriate for it does not 'fit' the present conditions of the hospitals with long waiting lists. With cold cases, for example, which become special during the consultation the patient-centred style can produce a dramatic anti-climatic effect at the end of the consultation. When a patient who has been made to feel very important and 'led to expect' special treatment then asks the gynaecologist for the date she will be admitted and he, being compelled to be realistic, replies, 'In nine to twelve months', the patient can now feel the proceedings have been tinged with 'deceit'. The gynaecologist is obliged to rectify the imbalance and renegotiate the relationship by bargaining over time with the patient. If the patient has a telephone, he will ask whether she is prepared to come in at very short notice, if another patient drops out, and so 'jump the queue'.

For the gynaecologist, time is a multiphase resource, which undergoes continuous matching exercises. He obviously has the commanding position in the regulation of hospital time. Patients do not have direct access to him as with the GP, which means he can manipulate time, *per se*, as a treatment component. The ductility of time in infertility cases, endowed with curative and diagnostic properties, is regarded as a manifestation of woman's 'biological naturalism'. The season of the year is also important. Christmas is traditionally a slack period for admissions and treatment. The old with no dependents can find their condition promoted to an urgent one and be invited to spend Christmas in hospital. The gynaecologist's calendar is becoming increasingly susceptible to instant revisions:[6] hospital militancy and financial stringency are but two recent factors.

The Reluctant Cancer Patient

In this final section, concerning a reluctant cancer patient, we have reproduced in some detail the talk by which the gynaecologist is forced to reveal the almost complete array of temporal antennae making up a gynaecological ideology. The temporal antennae are permutated and extended in an attempt to lock on to the patient's temporal framework and hence her source of meanings. Temporal projectioning is a major basis of the gynaecologist's authority. Some of the messages homing in on the patient are: A *short stay* in hospital is not socially disruptive. To be in an *early stage* of an illness is the ideal state. Illnesses have their temporal points of *no return*. There are *sensible* and *non sensible careers* in illness. To be ill is *wasting the time* of others. Treatment *prolongs* life. *Longevity* is beneficial. The *terminal* point of illness is the most unpleasant. *Night time* is a most *dangerous time* in a sickness career.

Gyn.: Right. I think I'll have to get you in fairly soon to examine you properly under an anaesthetic and take a sample from the neck of the womb.
P.: I don't want to come in.
Gyn.: You don't want to come in.
P,: No.
Gyn.: You won't be with us very long, just for two or three days. You see I think we ought to get a sample off the neck of the womb and I want the pathologist to have a look at it. And if it is what I think, I think we might have to send you to the Southern for some treatment.
P.: No, I don't want to go.
Gyn.: Yes.
P.: Do you think it is cancer?
Gyn.: Well, it might be.
P.: Oh . . . no.
Gyn.: Well, the point is you are here nice and early, aren't you?
P.: No.
Gyn.: The point is if you are here nice and early we can treat it. If you don't come in you are still going to have this discharge and bleeding. Aren't you?
P.: Are you sure?
Gyn.: Yes, but it is there. I have just done a smear now to take a few cells and it started bleeding again. The point is, if we get you in and get you treated we can cure it. Leave it another two or three months and it will be beyond curing it. I mean I'm not convinced one hundred per cent it is. I think it is. So we must make. . .
P.: Oh dear. I can't stand it.
Gyn.: Well, you will have to and you will have to come in.
P.: Cannot. [Sobs.]
Gyn.: You will have to. You have no choice.
P.: I wish I hadn't come.
Gyn.: Well I am glad you have come. I have a lady I went to see the other day, she had been bleeding at home for six months. Not only is she passing blood, but she is passing urine through the vagina. It's too late for me to do anything for her, because she has been silly and stayed at home. You have done just what you should have done. As soon as you had the slightest symptoms you

told the doctor. The doctor sent you to me without any delay, and I'm going to get you in here without any delay. I'll be sending for you with my next lot of patients. It won't be next week you will be coming in, it will probably be the Tuesday after.
P.: No, I can't leave my house.
Gyn.: Why can't you leave your house? Who's there?
P.: Nobody, only me.
Gyn.: Well, there is nobody to worry about. It is a House. It's a building isn't it?
P,: No I can't.
Gyn.: You must. What about your relatives? What relatives do you have in the area?
P,: I've got a son and my daughter is coming over from Canada.
Gyn.: When is she coming?
P.: Any time now.
Gyn.: Well, the point is we want to get you sorted out before she comes. Don't we? She doesn't want to go back thinking that she is wasting time to see her. You have no choice, You are coming in.
P.: Oh no. I'll go with it. I'll die with it.
Gyn.: You will be silly, you will be silly because you are what. . . Sixty. . . one. Now is it?
P.: Yes.
Gyn.: With treatment you are going to last till you are seventy-five. They will have to shoot you. At this stage it's a very early growth. [Softly.] It's very, *very*.
P.: I don't know why I have come.
Gyn.: But this is why you have come to me, to get it sorted out.
P.: Can I please myself?
Gyn.: You can please yourself, but I shall certainly chase you up. But if you don't do anything about it you are going to have a very nasty painful end. [Softly.] It will grow, you will start bleeding all the time. It will give rise to pain. It will extend into the bladder. You will finally become incontinent with urine and you may finally be incontinent with faeces. You may haemorrhage at night and they will bring you in and only the junior doctor will be there. And your family won't thank me for not chasing you up. You are as important to your family as well as to yourself, you know. So there is no doubt about it, you are coming in. Talk it over with the nurse if you want a lady to talk to. You will have to come in.

Discussion

The paper has portrayed some typical events occurring in the gynaecological consultation. The account has been systematically posed to show the significance of the temporal dimensions in the construction of the diagnostic order. It has been shown that there are many times, each with its own meanings and subsequent form of order, but all resonantly locked together. To identify but a few: chronological time, administrative time, documentary time, foetal time, historical time, reunion time, biological time, local time, seasonal time, pleasure time, disease time, menopause time and, not least, speaking time. These times interpenetrate, undergo mediation and protrude, 'appropriately', with emergent properties according to the rules in use.

By concentrating on speaking as performance, both the variability and the generality of activities in the gynaecological consultation have been picked out — this may, we hope, balance the Frankenstein creation of the generalised/statistical patient who is so frequently and robotically slotted into our 'higher theorising'. Although this study is male dominated and projected through the eyes of the gynaecologist, it does not mean that the patient is the dependent image. The ethnography of speaking accredits others with a rightful stance in the proceedings. In the last transcript the reluctant cancer patient's beliefs and motives were seen challenging successfully the might of the medical hierarchy. The patient and gynaecologist clashed; their respective segregates could not come to rest within the same taxonomies of time and space. The patient's reunion time consumed the gynaecologist's disease time; her house was more significant than a hospital (it certainly *wasn't* a building) in the ordering of events. Furthermore, there is no reason to believe that the category of reunion time (or house) is unequivocally linked to females, or their sexuality.

All those who enter into client relationships with the medical apparatus participate, to various degrees, in the rewriting of their histories. The rewriting of histories is an everyday feature of interaction. Gynaecology exaggerates this general medical and everyday activity, as we have shown, because of the uniqueness of its longitudinal involvements with women. Women more than men are engaged in restructuring their identities and creating new temporal significances for family, work, birth, menopause, fertility, etc. The study has explicated the interplay, constructs and movements between the various social times operative in the gynaecological consultation. Only by imposing crude typologies on the consultation will the clash between gynaecologist's time and women's time, as two discrete entities,

appear the only activity. Much of the reality of the situation will
also be negated if the encounter is translated solely into one of class
conflict. The same will ensue if women are caricatured as being
different from men because, according to Cottle's (1969) testing, they
are 'past-present orientaters'. (A view which can equate women with
manics, who are similarly dominated by the present.) In the consultation
we have shown that gynaecologist's and woman's time each fall under a
myriad of further self-categorisations, each of which has a different
episodic structure and each of which may be regarded as subjective
time. Even the quantitative aspect of administrative time manipulated
by the gynaecologist is in part a product of the social conventions of
others: the State and para- and non-medical unions are increasingly
involved in its definition and hence influence the consultation. A
patient may not wish to acknowledge an illness, like cancer, as
warranting a disturbance in a projection of social events. Another may
wish the gynaecologist to legitimate for her a new chronicling of events.
The medical trajectory of the patient provide both with forewarned
expectations. The administrative time for the session and the sequences
within each consultation produce their own concerns for temporal
ordering. We have shown how speech forms and speech events are
used not only to match and control the diagnostic sequencing but to
extract and convey, simultaneously, new temporal constructions
between the patient and gynaecologist. In routine cases strategies are
usually adopted to restrict the patient's history to the temporal horizon
of the 'strictly medically relevant'. With 'special' patients their histories
are often different in content and in their recounting. The social
contexting of their troubles within everyday events is more important.
'Special' patients possess openly more of their own histories and are
involved in a greater multiplicity of time. Patients can emerge as
'special' during the consultation. The patient with unusual connections
with the locality is but one instance. During the consultation she was
involved in 'time out' from the gynaecological interlude. Medical time
and lay time have many features of joint enterprise. They are derived
ultimately from the same font of collective experience.

Notes

1. For the sake of abbreviation we shall use throughout the term 'patient' in an unqualified way, acknowledging that many women are not ill, by any definition. Also, the consultants in question will be referred to as gynaecologists, although their functions overlap in the outpatient clinic with

2. some of their obstetric work.
   It is beyond the scope of this paper to elaborate the intricacies of a research partnership between a non-hospital-based sociologist and medical specialist. This study, one of a series being conducted within the obstetric/gynaecological orbit, is, as far as the sociologist is concerned, a preliminary examination of what can be regarded as 'moonrock' data. It is based on 207 consultations. Emerson's (1970) was based on 75, and Macintyre's on 55. Henslin's (1971) account was written in partnership with Biggs, an obstetric nurse, and was derived from 12-14,000 gynaecological examinations (only 2 refusals) over a 14-year period. It is not clear from the analysis whether Henslin was present as a non-participant observer.
3. Cassell (1976) raises a number of points relevant for gynaecology: how the doctor-patient language can be used to increase, or reduce, the distance between patient and disease. He reminds us that 'all treatments from poultices to renal dialysis are accompanied by words. We know much about the function of dialysis, but remarkably little about the function of words' (p. 146).
4. The position within a list can be significant. Some gynaecologists prefer their requests for terminations to be either at the beginning or the end. Some limit themselves to two per list, which means if one is added to the list it is more than likely one's request will be accepted, irrespective.
5. Gynaecologists recognise that their work can be seen to have a magico-religious significance. The patient's spatial progression to reach the 'inner sanctum' of the consultant is one aspect. Gynaecologists can offer no scientific explanations of why the 'same' treatment does not produce the same effect in the 'same' cases and thus evoke magic-type justifications. e.g. the patient's 'belief' in them. Sometimes this belief is deliberately cultivated to reinforce their technical skills, especially in unpredictable cases of women with repeated miscarriages who have to remain in hospital for five months or so before the baby is due.
6. During the hospital strike (Goldthorp and Richman, 1974b) the criteria of suitability for home delivery altered radically. Rh-negative mothers and primigravidae were delivered at home.

References

Baric, L. (1963), 'Some aspects of Credit, Saving and Investment in a "Non-Monetary" Economy', in R. Firth (ed.), *Capital Saving and Credit in Peasant Society* (Allen and Unwin, London).

Bauman, R. and Sherzer, J. (1974), *Exploration in the Ethnography of Speaking*, (Cambridge University Press).

Bauman, R. (1975), 'Verbal Art as Performance', *American Anthropologist* 77, pp. 290-311.

Ben-Sira, Z. (1976), 'The Function of the Professional's Affective Behaviour in Client Satisfaction: A Revised Approach to Social Interaction', *Journal of Health and Social Behaviour* 17, pp. 3-11.

Cassell, E. J., (1976), 'Disease as an "it": Concepts of Disease Revealed by Patients' Presentations of Symptoms', *Social Science and Medicine* 10, pp. 143-6.

Churchill, L. (1966), 'Notes on Everyday Quantitative Practices', paper presented to the methodological section of the American Sociological Association.

Cottle, J. T. (1969), 'Future Orientations and Avoidance: Speculations on the Time of Achievement and Social Roles', *The Sociological Quarterly*, pp. 419-37.

Emerson, J. (1970), 'Behaviour in Private Places: Sustaining Definitions of Reality in Gynaecological Examinations', in H. P. Dreitzel, *Recent Sociology No. 2 Patterns of Communicative Behaviour*, (Macmillan, New York, 1970), pp. 74-95.
Gluckman, M. (1964), *Closed Systems and Open Minds: the Limits of Naivety in Social Anthropology* (Edinburgh, Oliver and Boyd).
Goldthorp, W. O. and Richman, J. A. (1974a), 'The Gynaecological Patient's Knowledge of Her Illness and Treatment', A summary of the findings are produced in the *British Journal of Sexual Medicine*, Dec. 1975 and Feb. 1976.
Goldthorp W. O. and Richman J. A. (1974b), 'Maternal Attitudes to Unanticipated Home Confinement: A Case Study of the effects of the Hospital Strike upon Domiciliary Confinement', *Practitioner*, pp. 845-53.
Hayes-Bautista, D. E.(1976), 'The Termination of the Patient – Practitioner Relationships: Divorce, Patient Style', *Journal of Health and Social Behaviour* 17, pp. 12-21.
Henslin, J. and Biggs, M. (1971), 'Dramaturgical Desexualisation: the Sociology of the Vaginal Examination', in J. Henslin (ed.), *Studies in the Sociology of Sex* (Appleton-Century-Crofts, New York), pp. 243-72.
Hymes, D. (1962), 'The Ethnography of Speaking', in T. Gladwin (ed.), *Anthropology and Human Behaviour* (Anthropological Society of Washington) pp. 13-53.
Kaiser, B. L. and Kaiser, I. H. (1974), 'The Challenge of the Women's Movement to American Gynaecology', *Americal Journal of Obstetrics and Gynaecology* 120, pp. 652-665.
Katz, E., Gurevitch, M., Peled, T. and Danet, B. (1969), 'Doctor-Patient Exchanges: A Diagnostic Approach to Organizations and Professions', *Human Relations* 22, pp. 309-24.
Macintyre, S. (1976), 'To Have or to Have Not – Promotion and Prevention of Childbirth in Gynaecological Work', in M. Stacey (ed.), *The Sociology of the N.H.S.*, Sociological Review Monograph 22, pp. 176-93.
Manning, P. K. and Fabrega, H. (1973), 'The Experience of Self and Body: Health and Illness in the Chiapas Highlands', in G. Psathas (ed.), *Phenomenological Sociology: Issues and Applications* (John Wiley and Sons).
Reisman, K. (1974), 'Contrapuntal Conversations in an Antiguan Village', in Bauman, R., and Sherzer, J., op. cit.
Richman, J., Bedford, J. R. D. and Goldthorp, W. O. (1974), 'The Gynaecologist: Friend or Foe', *New Society* 30, pp. 474-6.
Scheflen, A. E. (1965), 'Quasi-Courting Behaviour in Psychotherapy', *Psychiatry*, 78, pp. 245-57.
Stimson, G. and Webb, B. (1975), *Going to See the Doctor. The Consultation Process in General Practice* (Routledge & Kegan Paul).
Sudnow, D. (1967), *Passing On: The Social Organization of Dying* (Prentice Hall, Inc., Englewood Cliffs, New Jersey).
Szasz, T. and Hollender, M. (1956), 'A Contribution to the Philosophy of Medicine: The Basic Models of the Doctor-Patient Relationship', *Archives of International Medicine* 97, pp. 585-92.
Turner, V. (1975), 'Dramas, Fields and Metaphors' (London, Cornell University Press).
Waitzkin, H. and Stoeckle, J.D. (1972), 'The Communication of Information about Illness', *Advanced Psychosomatic Medicine* 8, pp. 180-215.

It is interesting how many of the themes, including the disvaluing of patients' time, which have emerged in the preceding papers dealing with aspects of medical care in advanced industrial societies, are echoed in the study which follows by Cross and Arber of family planning in Trinidad and Tobago. Interesting, but not surprising since what they are studying is the introduction into the Carribean of a social policy devised in the advanced world and introduced through western medical organisation. This amounts to an imposition of particular practices and procedures upon clients who are not consulted but whose attitudes and behaviour are assumed. The reactions of the clients to this imposition are seen to be similar to reactions of clients in the West to policy makers and practitioners who do not consult them. Social, economic and cultural differences may be very considerable but the similarities of reaction are less surprising when one remembers that human beings are likely to react in essentially similar ways to relationships of subordination and domination wherever these may be found.

A conflict within the policy assumptions and between the rhetoric and the practice is found in these family planning clinics which echoes the conflict discussed by Mcintyre in an earlier paper. There the conflict was between, on the one hand, social policies for the elderly which were predominantly humanitarian in aim and which were directed to the individual needs of the elderly and, on the other hand, policies which were concerned to minimise the costs to the total society of the dependency of the elderly. In the paper that follows the conflict is between a rhetoric which stresses the benefits of family planning to the individual in terms of greater self-determination and a policy which appears to assume that population reduction is the goal. Clearly one cannot assume that greater self-determination will necessarily go along with a decline in number of children. Clearly, also, clients who believe that the family planning service is designed to increase their self-determination will expect a different service with a different emphasis from that which the organisers will offer if they are principally motivated to reduce the population. In the former case availability of contraception of a kind which the client finds acceptable when she wishes to avail herself of it is essential; in the latter case continuation of use of contraception at all times is likely to be the goal.

Cross and Arber show that the latter tends to dominate clinic practice. Women who discontinue clinic attendance are branded as dropouts whether they have stopped contracepting by choice to have a baby or for whatever reason. The presence of the conflict, and even more of the assumptions upon which the programme is based, are counterproductive in terms of both goals: the women do not necessarily get what they want when they want it; at the same time the programme could hardly be called a success in its own terms as the high incidence of discontinuation of attendance might indicate.

Cross and Arber make certain practical recommendations as a result of their survey. What they also do, as indeed do several others in this volume, is to raise the issue of conflict between professionals, their goals and practices, on the one hand and the aims of their patients or clients on the other. These conflicts reflect differing interests of different sections of the population. The differences are reflected in what is seen to be knowledge about a subject and how that knowledge is disseminated or translated into practice. The knowledge that is systematised is of course that of the organised professionals. The folk knowledge, the understanding of the people about their own situation, is less well articulated.

This and other papers in this book do not suggest definitive solutions to these conflicts. But before these can be found it is necessary that there should be an understanding of the partiality of professional knowledge and the consequences of that partiality for policy and practice.

M.S.

POLICY AND PRACTICE IN PARAMEDICAL ORGANISATIONS:
The Case of Family Planning Agencies

Malcolm Cross and Sara Arber

In a recent paper John Peel and Malcolm Potts lamented the lack of involvement of sociologists in research on family planning programmes (Peel and Potts, 1973). They attributed this to the continuing strength of anti-Malthusianism in sociology and the reluctance to accept that westerners had any right to interfere with the expansion of populations in underdeveloped countries. However, one can recognise the force of both these arguments and still be concerned about such programmes. Some £200 million is spent annually on providing clinics and contraceptives in the underdeveloped world and about half this amount comes from rich countries. This fact alone ought to guarantee critical attention, especially since the programmes are said to be 'ill conceived and sociologically unrealistic' (Peel and Potts, 1973, p. 184). In addition, it is widely and forcefully argued that access to effective contraception is a *sine qua non* of women's equality with men. For example, Lucinda Cisler has commented: 'Without the full capacity to limit her own reproduction, a woman's other "freedoms" are tantalizing mockeries that cannot be exercised. With it, the others cannot long be denied, since the chief rationale for denial disappears' (Cisler, 1970, p. 246).

Furthermore, it is possible to argue from a non-Malthusian viewpoint that personal control over fertility for both sexes is an act of awareness which may instigate greater concern for wider political issues. Although Ivan Illich may have changed his earlier views, since hormonal contraception has clear iatrogenic effects, he has made a powerful plea for considering education in contraception as having an inter-dependent relationship with political awareness and community participation. Thus the realisation that sex need not produce an unwanted pregnancy 'provokes another concept: the insight that economic survival does not have to breed political exploitation', while 'education in modern parenthood could become a powerful form of agitation to help an uprooted mass grow into "people" ' (Illich, 1973, pp. 119, 128).

The policies of international agencies project ideological assumptions about family planning. In this paper we examine some of those assumptions and compare them with the experience of 'clients' in one programme in the Commonwealth Caribbean. The data for this exercise come from a study carried out by the authors in 1975 into the problem of clinic discontinuation.[1]

Policy and Practice

There is an important and interesting conflict in the declared policy of family planners, particularly at the level of international agencies. On the one hand, organisations like the International Planned Parenthood Federation (IPPF) declare themselves to have as their main emphasis 'the spread of ideas which will permit and encourage men and women everywhere to make informed decisions about having children' (Macdonald, 1973, p. 3). If this is the dominant ideology it follows that an assessment of changes in fertility rates can have little to do with evaluating programmes, unless it can be shown that people actually want less children than they have or expect to have. On the other hand, the whole tenor of debate, and most of the reviews and evaluations of family planning programmes, concern a decline in birthrate. The difference would not in itself be of great interest were it not for the fact that the attempt to rationalise the latter policy by making it compatible with the liberal sentiments of the former has produced one of the main strands in research so far — the knowledge, attitudes and practice (KAP) surveys (cf. Berelson, 1966). This is turn has had a profound effect upon the policies which have been used to demonstrate unmet need. It is indoubtedly true, as Coser has recently reminded us, that modern research methods can influence our choice of problem, and may thus serve to widen the gulf between problem and theory (Coser, 1975). Equally, however, choice of research method (as in KAP surveys) may depend upon ideology and may then produce results that serve to legitimate predetermined policies.

Despite the attempts to present family planning as an opportunity for informed decision-making, there is no doubt that Malthusian fears of the implications of uncontrolled population growth are dominant in family planning movements. This is not necessarily on the grounds of some apocalyptic vision but simply because population growth is perceived as inhibiting development. But how is fertility to be checked? As Burch (1975) has pointed out, the more sophisticated multi-causality theories of fertility decline are very hard to put into practice. The tendency has been to adhere to more simplistic notions based upon premises of technical adequacy and 'rationalism' (that if people have knowledge of contraception, they will wish to practice it).

Policy and Practice in Paramedical Organisations

It follows from these premises that supply, information and education are the three major elements to successful population control policies. Alternative views have either tended to argue that smaller families are likely to be a consequence of economic development or that the family planning approach fails to understand the complexities of male-female interaction, the subordinate status of women, and the social and psychological role of children. A good example of the first view is given by William Rich (1973) when he concludes, on the basis of a survey of a dozen countries, that 'development policies that focus on participation and increased access to benefits for the population as a whole do seem to produce a major impact on family size' (Rich, 1973, p. 37). The other view concentrates on the very important question of motivation. It points to the fact that if procreation provides institutionalised rewards then this, more than ideals, can provide ample motivation for child bearing. As Judith Blake puts it:

> Children are high on the list of adult utilities. Offspring are not simply outlets (and inlets) for affection, they are the instrumentalities for achieving virtually prescribed social statuses ('mother' and 'father'), the almost exclusive avenues for feminine creativity and achievement... until nonfamilial roles begin to offer significant competition to familial ones as avenues for adult satisfaction, the family will probably continue to amaze us with its procreative powers. (Blake, 1965 quoted in Scanzoni and Murray, 1972, p. 318.)

It is, of course, true that these two perspectives are 'beyond family planning' but they have to be borne in mind in evaluating the 'success' of programmes of fertility control since changes in either could cause a spurious correlation between availability of programmes and declines in age-specific fertility.

Even the defenders of family planning programmes are unlikely to state unequivocally that the causal line is clear. There is considerable evidence that many declines started *before* family planning programmes. As Philip Hauser points out (1970) even the 'successful' programmes in Taiwan, Hong Kong, Singapore and South Korea have to be seen in the context of rising income and education levels which appear to have influenced fertility before specific programmes were introduced. Similarly any assessment of effectiveness has to take account of changes in the age of marriage and of the proportion married.

There is then evidence to suggest that the 'campaign for population control is going badly' (Peel and Potts, 1973, p. 184) if one means by this lack of evidence that such programmes are having an independent effect on fertility patterns. It would be foolish to deny that such massive resources must be producing some consequence, but the evidence that they have achieved in practice what they set out to achieve, if one takes this to be a decline in age-specific fertility, has yet to be satisfactorily adduced.

Ideology and Family Planning

We will examine the reasons for this lack of 'success' of family planning programmes in terms of the various assumptions made within the family planning movement about the behaviour of individuals and the appropriate mode of disseminating family planning advice and materials. The origin of these assumptions that form a core part of the ideology of family planning are not our main focus in this paper.

We suggest that there are four basic elements to the dominant ideology which can be found in most family planning programmes. These will be illustrated by relating them to the problem of clinic discontinuation. The general ideology provides us with assumptions that provide expectations, which can be examined in relation to the Trinidad data.

The four elements of ideology are expressed here as basic assumptions:

1. The assumption of method acceptability.
2. The assumption of simple rationality.
3. The assumption of clinic distribution.
4. The assumption of the hegemony of doctors.

1. The Assumption of Method Acceptability

According to this perspective the problem of family planning is mainly one of method acceptability. KAP studies repeatedly show 'high interest in learning' about birth control and, indeed, usually considerable knowledge of some available methods. The problem is conceptualised as how to deliver the most acceptable method. Fifty-nine per cent of the US Agency for International Development's research monies is spent on the development of contraceptive methods that will be more effective, not simply in the sense of take-up, but also reliability in use (use effectiveness) and use over time (extended use effectiveness) (cf. Bone, 1975; Tietze, 1970). Critics of this line of reasoning point out that it drastically oversimplifies the motivation issue. It is said to reduce the motive problem 'to a technological question. The task of population control then becomes simply the invention of a device that will be acceptable.' (Davis, 1970a, p. 377.) Others suggest that it has an inherently conservative flavour since it presumes that no other social or political transformation is required. Therefore programmes based on this assumption are thought likely to prove acceptable to conventional elites. As Kenneth Godwin suggests: 'By implying that the only need is the invention and distribution of new technological devices, family planning programmes do not disturb the elites and are therefore more readily accepted by the host society.' (Godwin, 1973, p. 136.) The fundamental question 'what population policy is best?' is not therefore asked. Instead this aspect of the dominant ideology only permits the question 'how can we improve the effectiveness of family planning programmes?'.

2. The Assumption of Simple Rationality

The KAP studies referred to earlier are largely concerned to discover attitudes and opinions, as well as knowledge and practice, of birth control. If such studies are to be used for policy purposes then the assumption has to be made that a relationship exists between attitudes and behaviour such that information on the strength or direction of attitudes can predict variations in the behaviour. It is perhaps here more than anywhere else that the lack of a basic sociological focus to such studies is clear. In the first place there are serious doubts expressed about the research techniques employed in KAP studies (Cleland, 1973; Godwin, 1972) but also there is little reason to suppose that attitudes are highly predictive of behaviour, particularly in areas where emotion and affectivity are involved (cf. La Pierre, 1934). For example, Philip Hauser has stressed that KAP surveys often show a 70 per cent 'interest in learning' about birth control but only 7-10 per cent acceptor rate. As he continues: 'This gap certainly raises serious questions about the validity of the survey response and the assumption of rational behaviour.' (Hauser, 1970, p. 357.)

The point is that other variables intervene between a predisposition to act and action itself. The attitudes of others, for example, may be relevant or the structural features of the situation such as cost or, in the case of free facilities, the ease with which a woman may reach a distribution point. G. A. Viestra put it well when he stressed that take up of services, even when attitudes are favourable, may include:

... the staunch aversion against any form of contraception her husband possesses or the vehement disapproval of reference groups and persons, frightening rumours, the expense of the contraceptive, the trouble she must go to in order to reach the family planning clinic or her fear of the male doctor she will find once she gets there. (Viestra, 1974, pp. 22-3.)

Variables such as these may form part of a response to a situation which is characterised by 'rationality', but not in the simple form that equates attitudes concerning a specified object with action taken in relation to it.

In assessing the reasons for discontinuation both the assumptions we have discussed could be important. They have in common the fact that they direct attention towards the clients, either in their response to a particular method or in terms of their attitudes to contraceptive use. Investigation of the other two assumptions directs the researcher's attention towards the family planning programme itself; they do not therefore tend to be seen as problematic by defenders of such programmes.

3. The Assumption of Clinic Distribution

This refers to the fact that the most appropriate method of contraceptive distribution is seen as being one where the clients attend a local organisation such as a clinic or health centre. There may be problems with their location, opening times and the fact that many women are often expected to wait for very long periods to see a nurse or doctor. Peel and Potts point to this problem when they refer to the 'inconvenient siting of clinics, inconvenient opening hours, delays and embarrassing examinations and questioning' (Peel and Potts, 1973, p. 185).

The clinic organisation can also make the use of family planning known to one's friends and neighbours. It is likely that some women travel longer distances than necessary to mask their attendance. The embarrassment at using contraception is a factor to consider, as is the possible stigma that attaches to being seen to need to limit the size of one's family. This is something that will vary in strength from one culture to another but J. R. van Renselaar, in an anthropological study of a Tunisian village, found that:

> ... adopting birth control measures is apparently considered public acknowledgement of poverty. It is therefore not done. The stigma of indigence constitutes a significant barrier to modern birth control.

We can even ask ourselves to what extent medical dangers cited as objections to birth control should be interpreted as a rationalization disguising a reluctance to publicly avow poverty. (van Renselaar, 1974, p. 71.)

We should be sensitive therefore to the possibility that factors related to the administration and organisation of clinics may be relevant to retaining clinic attenders.

4. The Assumption of the Hegemony of Doctors

The prevalence of clinic organisation is in itself testimony to the primacy of the medical model and the role of the medical profession. It is based on the supposition that fertility control by contraception is a branch of preventive medicine. The integration of clinics into antenatal and child welfare services is further evidence of this, as is the role of the physician as an arbiter of appropriate contraceptive technique.

Although the status of doctors may have been useful in order to obtain approval from national governments and religious organisations for family planning, it is sometimes suggested that the profession may be a constraining rather than a promoting force. Peel and Potts write: 'For several methods outlets are controlled by a powerful and long established trade union — the medical profession — which until recently condemned all methods of family planning and many branches of which still refuse certain essential options.' (Peel and Potts, 1973, p. 185.)

There are often very few doctors in poor countries so that their role as gatekeepers has an even more limiting effect on access to family planning. Also the very association with doctors may confirm in the eyes of some the dangers to health inherent in contraception. Even in the UK it has been suggested that consultations and examinations should be kept to a minimum on the grounds that 'possibly the most important reason why the poor, ill-educated and underprivileged fail to use contraception may well be the need to consult professionals whose authoritarian image inhibits them' (Diggory and McEwan, 1976, 93). It has also been pointed out that although women are medically examined before the pill is prescribed, they are not before conception, although the risks are greater (Potts, 1971). Although some danger of thromboembolism may exist with pill use, doctors cannot predict who is at risk aside from enquiries about varicose veins or phlebitis — which can and are made by paramedical staff in many countries (see Kerr, 1972).

The medical model also entails gaining access to the clinics and doctors, which can be a very time-consuming process. Feminist critiques have suggested that if you walk into the waiting-room of an obstetric clinic in the United States 'you will see it full of women waiting patiently to be called . . . they are victims in the gynaecologist's waiting room . . . of the assumption that a woman's time is of no value' (Kaiser and Kaiser, 1974, p. 657). The same view often asserts that male doctors in particular fail to acknowledge the right of a woman to know about her own body, or mystify the simplest procedures, or sacrifice the time and comfort of patients to their own convenience (cf. Muller, 1974, p. 70).

The Problem of Discontinuation

Overall, these four assumptions do combine to form a distinct stance on the question of family planning programmes; they comprise a coherent ideological position that has determined most policy responses. In examining a situation where some women have apparently rejected family planning services it is possible to compare those who continue with those who 'drop-out' in relation to these four assumptions. The clinics themselves will tend to perceive the 'problem' of the gap between the policy of maintaining users of their services and the practice of losing a substantial number, in terms of their clients. The very term 'drop-out', which is commonly used to label discontinuers, suggests the perceived locus of explanation. The 'drop-out' is different in that she actively rejects, rather than being the recipient of rejection by others. Our discussion so far enables us to appreciate that this may be only part of the process. If the critiques of the medical model and clinic programmes are to be believed then one might presume that 'clinic' factors have some explanatory weight. Although each element can break down into a number of propositions, if we take the position of the dominant ideology in family planning then the following proposals should hold:

> If the problem is one of method acceptability then discontinuation would be higher from the least acceptable method.
> If the problem is one of attitude then discontinuation would be associated with negative attitudes towards family planning.
> If clinic based services are unproblematic then discontinuation will not be associated with waiting time and other experiences of clinic services.
> If the role of doctors is unexceptionable then discontinuation will not be associated with a negative experience of their services.

Policy and Practice in Paramedical Organisations

It is important to note that we have preferred the term 'discontinuer' to 'drop-out' since the former describes behaviour without attributing causation. The label 'drop-out', like the expression 'defaulter' to identify non-compliance with doctors' orders, clearly locates the blame for the behaviour with the client or patient (cf. Stimson, 1974). This is also an ideological manifestation since once the assumption is made that the client is at fault, the obvious research task is to investigate the characteristics of the deviant and not the institutional and organisational processes that underlie the application of the label.

Fertility and Family Planning in Trinidad and Tobago

In the Caribbean as a whole, the rate of population growth is high; indeed for the period 1950-70 it has been estimated at 3 per cent per annum which is only slightly less than Central America, the fastest in the world (Segal, 1974, p. 8). The picture is, however, highly variable with considerable differences both within the Commonwealth Caribbean and between it and the rest. Between 1960 and 1970 the population of the Dominican Republic grew by 42.5 per cent, Cuba by 26.9 per cent and Guyana by 24.8 per cent, while Jamaica and Trinidad and Tobago at 10.3 per cent and 12.4 per cent respectively had averages around the Commonwealth Caribbean norm of 12.7 per cent (Davis, 1970b, Table A; Commonwealth Caribbean, 1974).

The crude birth-rate in Trinidad and Tobago dipped below 35 in 1964 and continued to decline to reach a low of 24.5 in 1969. It subsequently climbed to 26.8 in 1972 and fell again to 24.7 in 1973. (Trinidad and Tobago, 1975, p. 2), although there is a possibility that this was a spurious increase produced by under-enumeration in the 1970 Census (total population just over 1 million). There is evidence to show that the decline in the 1960s was produced by a reduction on fertility rather than by changes in the age composition of the population (Mandle, 1973, p. 3). Younger women appear to have initiated the fertility decline (Trinidad and Tobago, 1974b, p. 31), particularly those in non-legal ('common-law' or 'visiting') unions. However, there is no conclusive evidence that this was the result of family planning programmes, or even of contraceptive use, although Trinidad is often cited in the same breath as Taiwan as a 'successful' location.

The population of Trinidad and Tobago is racially varied; 43 per cent is African in origin, 40 per cent Asian and 14 per cent is classified in the Census as 'mixed' (black/white). White, Chinese and those of Syrian and Lebanese extraction comprise the remainder. The population is unevenly distributed in racial terms with Africans predominating in most urban areas and northern counties, while Indians form a majority in the rural areas of the central and south of the island. It is generally recognised that age-specific fertility rates for the Indian population are higher than for the other groups although no recent rates are available. The 1970 Census recorded that 32 per cent of African women between 15 and 44 years of age had three or more children, compared with 44 per cent of Indian women in the same age group (Trinidad and Tobago, 1974c, Table 6).

Trinidad is relatively rich by Third World standards; indeed in the last four years the expansion of the oil industry has effectively removed the island from the ranks of undeveloped countries in terms of *per capita* income. This comparative affluence is likely to have had its effect on recent fertility declines (cf. Freedman and Berelson, 1976).

There has been a rapid growth in the number of family planning clinics since the first clinic was started by expatriate volunteers in 1956. The total number of clinics in operation in 1968 was 17 and by 1970 this had risen to 37. By the end of 1975, there were 72 clinics sponsored by the Government issuing free contraceptives; 47 of these are integrated with other health services and 9 are exclusively male centres. In addition the Family Planning Association (FPA) runs 5 clinics which are not integrated with any other services, and there is one clinic sponsored by the Catholic Marriage Advisory Council. Relatively few pronouncements about the demographic targets of the National Family Planning Programme have been made apart from at the establishment of the Population Council in 1967, which had the stated purpose of co-ordinating a national policy to reduce the birth-rate to 19 by 1977 (Harewood, 1968, pp. 885-7; Andrews, 1975, pp. 73-87: Harewood and Abdullah, 1971, pp. 4-7).

It is hard to arrive at a genuine figure for the proportion of new attenders who subsequently discontinue clinic attendance. The director of the Government Programme puts the total discontinuation rate at 34 per cent of the clients registered in 1972 (Andrews, 1975, p. 79). She estimates that there were approximately 31,000 current users in 1972 and the Report on the Population Programme for 1973 puts the figure at 34,508, or 32 per cent of the target population (which is half the female population between the ages of 15 and 44) (Trinidad and Tobago, 1974a, p. 9). We have estimated the total number of attenders in 1974 to be approximately 42,000, of which 47 per cent attended the five FPA clinics. The FPA gave its discontinuers as 7,941 in 1974, which represents 28.8 per cent of clients for that year (Family Planning Association, 1975, p. 14). From the figures we obtained we estimate the

1974 discontinuation rate for FPA clinics and government clinics to be 33 per cent and 44 per cent respectively.[2] The high rates of discontinuation mask the fact that at least 50 per cent of those who are defined as 'drop-outs' by the clinics will subsequently re-attend a family planning clinic. In fact, for the FPA, 5,913 clients were defined as 'restarters' in the programme in 1974 compared with 7,941 who were defined as 'discontinuers' (Family Planning Association, 1975, p. 15).

1975 Trinidad Survey

Our sample consists of 1,050 women interviewed in their own homes by female Trinidadian interviewers between September and November 1975. There is enormous variability in the family planning clinics themselves, particularly in relation to size (measured in annual number of attenders) but also in the number of times they are open each week and other structural and locational characteristics. The small clinics tend to be run by the Government in rural or semi-urban areas and most of them are integrated with other health services, whereas the large clinics are mostly urban and have sessions run separately from other health services (4 out of the 5 FPA clinics fall into this category). Our sample of women was designed to represent clinic types and not the population of clinic attenders. A purposive sample of 13 clinics was selected to represent these various types of clinic.[3]

The definition of a 'drop-out' used by the clinics, and in the sample, is a client who has not returned to the clinic for three calendar months after the month she was scheduled to return. This definition is used for women on all family planning methods except the IUD, who were excluded from this study.[4] The discontinuers selected from each clinic were a random sample of women who should have returned in the six months before 1 June 1975 and who had not returned by early September. The sample of 'continuers' from each clinic was matched with the discontinuer sample to control for length of clinic registration.[5] The sample was weighted in favour of discontinuers to continuers in the ratio 60:40, resulting in a final sample containing 617 discontinuers and 433 continuers; response rates of 74 per cent and 80 per cent respectively.

There are a number of different ways of delineating the groups in our sample. We may, for example, define discontinuers as those who are labelled 'drop-outs' by the clinics or we may prefer self-categorisation either in terms of stated attendance within the previous four months or of intention to return by some designated date in the future. The meaning of clinic discontinuation varies; some may discontinue all methods while others merely stop going to the clinics, obtaining their supplies of the same or a different method from other sources. In this analysis we have contented ourselves with the clinic labels but drawn a distinction between those who stop all use of contraceptives (Methdisc) and those who cease attending the clinic but still use a birth control method (Clindisc). The reason for this latter distinction is partly because those who discontinue all methods include a significant proportion who are planning their families and have decided to try to become pregnant while the other group are, from the clinic's point of view, a more serious problem since their continued use of contraception suggests the maintenance of motivation. Continuers are defined as those maintaining both method use and clinic attendance.

1. Method Acceptability

The assumption of method acceptability implies that the more reliable contraceptive devices will be most acceptable to the client. The implicit assumption is that technologically efficient methods without side-effects can act as a substitute for weak motivation to have less children. The majority of family planning programmes sees the pill and IUD as the most reliable and easy to use methods, and therefore assume that if women can be persuaded to use these methods there will be less necessity for a powerful desire to limit family size.

We will first examine the proposition of method acceptability in relation to the pill and later to condoms and foams or creams (as mentioned earlier clients currently using the IUD were excluded from this study). A very high proportion, 86 per cent, of the total sample have used the pill at some time, although only 58 per cent of those still using a method were using the pill at the time of the interview. The conclusion emerges from these data that the pill is unacceptable to many women. The main reasons women gave for discontinuing pill use are analysed in Table 1. For women no longer using a method and for those now using some other method, the most important stated reason for discontinuing the pill is side-effects, given by 42 per cent and 78 per cent respectively. Side-effects were coded when a respondent mentioned experiencing a health problem which she thought was caused by taking the pill.

The role of side-effects in leading to discontinuation of pill and birth control usage is illustrated in Table 2; of those who say they have experienced no side-effects 60 per cent are still using the pill. The proportion still using the pill decreases to 17 per cent for those reporting three or more side-effects. Some of the women no longer using the pill

Table 1. Main Reason for Discontinuation of Pill Use: (a) For women no longer using a method who used the pill as their last method; (b) For women currently using a method who used the pill as their previous method (per cent).

Reasons for Discontinuation	(a) No longer using birth control	(b) Still using birth control
Desired pregnancy	13	1
Pregnant while using pill	11	4
No need/illness	16	5
Side-effects	42	78
Fear about method	1	2
Problem with supplies	4	2
Other reasons	13	8
	100%	100%
	(287)	(163)

Table 2. Number of Side Effects Experienced by Sometime Users of the Pill by Current Family Planning Use (per cent).

	Number of Side Effects				
	0	1	2	3 or more	Total
Still using pill	60	32	22	17	39
Using a method other than pill	7	22	35	30	20
Using no method	33	46	43	52	41
	100	100	100	100	100
	(328)	(305)	(202)	(69)	(904)

are using another method, but in each case a larger proportion discontinue all contraceptive practice. This may be a negative impact of pill use, if a woman is then discouraged from using any other method because of her experience with the pill, or because of the lack of realistic alternative methods offered by the clinic programme. However, the pill may be the ideal method of family planning where side-effects are minimal, since there is a higher satisfaction among current pill users than among any other group: 77 per cent of women using the pill are completely satisfied with that method, compared with 64 per cent using condoms and 55 per cent using foam or cream.

An alternative question relating to method acceptability is whether particular methods lead to greater discontinuation of clinic attendance and family planning use. This is difficult to answer because of the variety and complexity of contraceptive histories (e.g. condoms may be the most recent method given to a client because of side-effects or contraindication to use of the pill, but not the method of first choice).

Women currently using condoms or foam are more experienced contraceptors, since 79 per cent of the former and 90 per cent of the latter have used some other method of family planning compared with only 27 per cent of women currently using the pill. Subsequent discontinuation may be examined in terms of the last method given by the clinic (see Table 3). Fewer of those who discontinue were last given the pill and more either foam or no method. Equivalent proportions of those who discontinue use of all methods and those who continue to attend the clinics were given condoms, 17-18 per cent. However, a substantially greater proportion of women who discontinue

Table 3. Continuer Status by Method Reported as Last Given by Family Planning Clinic (per cent).

	Methdisc	Clindisc	Continuer	Total
Pill	59	42	74	60
Condom	18	29	17	20
Foam/Cream	10	10	3	8
Other Methods	3	9	1	4
No Method Given	10	10	5	8
	100	100	100	100
	(445)	(235)	(368)	(1048)

clinic use but continue to use some method were last given condoms, 29 per cent. This suggests that use of condoms is not a cause of family planning discontinuation, but that for condom users the clinics may not be such an essential or the most appropriate source of supply.

The assumption of method acceptability implicitly supported by most family planners is too simplistic; a single technologically efficient method will not be acceptable to all women motivated to limit their family size. Discontinuation might decline if more emphasis is placed on the diversity of methods available and a realistic choice of methods is given to clients instead of the current pro-pill policy.

2. Simple Rationality

The basic assumption underlying the use of the results of KAP surveys as a justification for instituting and supporting family planning programmes, is that women say they have, or expect to have, more children than they want. If this assumption is true, one would expect that those continuing with family planning would be those who want no more children. This is not borne out by the Trinidad data, which show that 72 per cent of women who have discontinued all family planning use (Methdisc) say they do not want any more children, compared with 71 per cent of those who have only discontinued clinic attendance (Clindisc) and 70 per cent of Continuers. Similarly, it was found that 61 per cent did not want to have another child at the time they were pregnant with their last child, which also does not vary between categories of client. The findings imply that whether a woman wants more children or wanted her last child has no effect on the continuity of clinic attendance.

Other factors, apart from the stated attitudes of the client, are clearly important intervening variables between her attitudes and contraceptive behaviour — for example, the attitudes of her partner towards family planning. Where these are more favourable it is more likely that the client will continue both clinic attendance and birth control usage; this is shown by the data in Table 4. Sixty-seven per cent of those who discontinue using family planning state that they have partners who strongly agree with its use compared with 88 per cent for 'continuers'.

Although the woman's desire for more children does not affect her likelihood of discontinuation, the partner's reported desire for additional children has a more substantial influence. Of those who discontinue all family planning (Methdisc) 46 per cent have partners who want more children compared with only 34 per cent of those

Table 4. Continuer Status by Reported Partner's Attitude to Respondent Using Family Planning (per cent).

	Methdisc	Clindisc	Continuer	All
Strongly Agrees	67	82	88	79
Agrees a little	16	10	7	11
Doesn't mind	4	4	2	3
Disagrees	13	4	3	7
	100	100	100	100
	(327)	(225)	(356)	(909)

using family planning obtained from sources other than clinics (Clindisc), and 38 per cent of those who continue clinic use. One can hypothesise that the partner's attitudes have some influence on a woman's contraceptive behaviour irrespective of her desires for more children. The second hypothesis of simple rationality is not supported, since a client's stated desire for no more children is unrelated to her subsequent contraceptive behaviour.

3. Clinic Distribution

There is evidence from the survey results that attending the clinic posed problems associated with discontinuation, for example, those who maintained contraceptive use but discontinued attending the clinics were more likely to live further away and to travel to the clinics by taxi. On the whole it took them longer to reach the clinics although there was no evidence that financial factors lay behind their decision to stop attending.

Most visits to the clinics are for supplies. A majority of our respondents waited less than forty minutes for their supplies but nearly 20 per cent actually waited for more than an hour. Those who discontinued did not report being any worse off in this regard. It is suspected that the ease of obtaining these supplies from other sources is a strong factor in producing clinic discontinuation. In addition nearly all the clinics visited indicated that condoms were in short supply and often clinics only received a small proportion of their monthly orders. As a result many were only able to supply a small number and would often tell their clients to return or, indeed, to buy their supplies. In some cases clients were advised to take the pill for a month rather than have no protection! We suspect that a number of those told to return actually bought alternative supplies or used nothing since, in addition to waiting and travelling time, condom usage can be seen as an embarrassing index of sexual activity. Lack of supplies appears to be related to clinic discontinuation, since 28 per cent of clinic discontinuers reported that either suppliers of their last method or pill brand were not always available compared to 17 per cent of continuers. It is worth stressing that the shortage of condoms appeared to be so ubiquitous as to be a deliberate policy. This is, of course, entirely in line with the medical model since condoms, not being drugs, are thought less appropriate for clinic distribution.

Table 5. Privacy in Clinics by Continuer Status

Per cent replying not enough privacy when:

	Methdisc	Clindisc	Continuer	All
Getting supplies	15	22	15	16(1020)
Changing and undressing	15	24	20	19 (968)
Being examined and fitted	12	23	16	16 (925)

As Table 5 shows, clinic discontinuers were more likely to complain about a lack of privacy in the clinics. Accommodation would often be very rudimentary with makeshift buildings, which, together with the need to maintain a cooling breeze, ensure that little that passed between nurse and client remained private. A number of nurses pointed out the constraining effects of poor accommodation. One claimed that humour was her way of overcoming the tensions created by lack of privacy, another that she had to take clients to a garage at the side of the main building in order to discuss particularly personal problems, such as loss of libido or other sexual problems. Accommodation difficulties and overcrowding were one of the main reasons why most nurses in the clinics were lukewarm about the logical extension of the preventive health model: the integration of family planning with (other) health services. Others pointed out that the service was entirely different, requiring more advice and help, or that holding family planning and child welfare or antenatal clinics on the same day was counter-productive since the presence of young children advertised the attractions of motherhood!

We were particularly interested in the stigmatising effect of being a returned discontinuer. Most women at one time or another are labelled as 'drop-outs' and when this occurs their files are often removed from the main register. This immediately identifies them on their return and they are frequently left in little doubt that 'dropping-out', for whatever reason, is strongly to be deprecated. The semi-public situation in which the interaction between nurse and client occurs magnifies its negative effect. Instances were observed of women returning to the clinics who were questioned loudly by counter staff about their reasons for not coming back before in front of clients who were waiting to be seen. In one such instance the nurse, after being unable to find the client's case card in the current files, stated 'You're a drop-out'. The woman was then left standing while the nurse saw to other clients who were waiting at the counter. After about ten minutes, the returned 'drop-out' was asked 'What happened? You have a baby?' The client gave a muffled embarrassed explanation which could not be heard by the rest of the clients waiting, at which the nurse concluded in a loud voice 'You didn't have sex, then?'.

We asked our respondents whether the clinic staff had treated them 'harshly' (a word which in Trinidad carries a connotation of bureaucratic insensitivity). Table 6 suggests that those who still continue family planning but who stop going to the clinics are twice as likely to report experiences of 'harsh' treatment by both nurses and counter staff (sometimes one and the same).

Table 6. Proportion of Respondents Who Claimed That Clinic Staff Had Treated Them 'Harshly' by Continuer Status (per cent)

Staff	Continuer Status			
	Methdisc	Clindisc	Continuer	All
Counter Staff	10	15	8	10(1040)
Nurses	10	17	8	11(1040)

We suspect that in a society where class, education and gender conspire to produce low levels of confidence in the face of bureaucracy these figures underestimate the amount of negative clinic experience. An additional factor resulting in such underestimation is the reactivity of the interview situation, in which the middle-class interviewers were

Policy and Practice in Paramedical Organisations

often seen by the respondents as representatives of the clinic. However, there are grounds for rejecting the third hypothesis; discontinuation does appear to be related to clinic services.

4. The Role of Doctors

Each client is expected to see a doctor on registering with the clinic and annually or more frequently if she experiences any problems that require medical attention. However, many of the doctors working in government family planning clinics have no training in family planning. For example, clients may have to go to another clinic to have an IUD or diaphragm fitted, or a nurse may have to do the PAP smear tests. In these clinics it is still seen as necessary for the client to be examined by the doctor even though the doctor may only be able to do a pelvic examination and not the other procedures associated with family planning care.

From visiting more than twenty clinics, interviewing staff and observing them in operation, it is quite clear that doctors are instrumental in wasting the time of clients. In a considerable number of cases doctors simply did not show up for the sessions (usually meant to be three hours) for which they were paid, leaving considerable numbers of women waiting to no avail from 8.30 in the morning until lunch time. In one case, for example, the District Medical Officer was due one day a week at 9 a.m. but by 12.15 had not arrived and we were told that he 'sometimes only comes once a month'. On other occasions approximately half the women had gone home by the time the doctor arrived.

The doctor-client relationship in the clinics was of the most superficial kind. The time each woman spent with the doctor could be measured in seconds rather than minutes (we observed a case where 34 women received internal examinations in 25 minutes — including 4 IUD insertions and prescriptions for 3 cases of pelvic inflammatory disease!). This rapid turnover existed even where the doctor was only an hour late and appears to be a result of the low status that family planning has within the medical profession. This, and the conflict engendered by lucrative private practice, seems to account for the problems that we noted in the majority of clinics. The status of doctors, together with the fact that most of them are men in a world where the majority of clients and staff are women, ensures that this situation is seldom brought to the attention of the authorities. In a number of cases, nurses in charge would spend considerable time preparing their clients, both physically and psychologically, for rapid examination.

There was much evidence of a deep concern by nurses for the well-being of their clients, to the extent of giving supplies at non-family planning clinic times for the convenience of the client and taking supplies to the client while the District Nurse was on her domiciliary rounds. These practices were against the regulations of the official programme, which often appeared to be more concerned with maintaining accurate clinic records than providing a service to the consumer.

The problem of waiting time before seeing a doctor is reflected in our respondents' replies. Overall 60 per cent had waited more than two hours. We also asked people about how annoyed they felt at these delays; 27 per cent overall recorded annoyance, which was more than twice the proportion expressing such feelings about other clinic services. However, these findings do not discriminate between different categories of continuers. Dissatisfaction was shown by clients and especially by nurses about the actions of doctors in the family planning programme. Some nurses specifically mentioned that 'doctors are too interested in their private practices'. Our conclusion that doctors hold a too central role in the Trinidad family planning programme is derived largely from our observational material where clients were seen to 'vote with their feet' and from unfocused interviews with nurses, not from a finding of greater stated dissatisfaction with doctors among those who discontinued clinic use.

Conclusion

The emphasis of family planing programmes in underdeveloped countries, particularly those supported by international agencies, promotes the use of more reliable, female-centred methods of birth control under the auspices of health-related organisations. It is explicitly stated that the policy goal in the Trinidad case, in common with many programmes elsewhere, is not to *control* populations but to enable people to plan their families in line with their preferred family size. However, anyone not returning to the clinic after a specified period is labelled by the clinic staff, and enters into the clinic records, by the perjorative term 'drop-out'. If the programme was fulfilling its goal of allowing women to *plan* their families a proportion would discontinue attendance because they desire to have a child, no longer need to use family planning, or because of illness. Twenty-eight per cent of the reasons given by respondents for not returning to the clinic in this study can be classified as reasons that would be 'legitimate' in terms of official aims, yet they are all labelled 'drop-outs'. We are drawn to the

Policy and Practice in Paramedical Organisations

conclusion that the programme is orientated towards the *control* of family size.

In practice the attempt has been made to deliver the technically most effective method but we have not been able to show that this is universally preferred. Rather, it appears as if genuine choice of method, including those that are less reliable or less technically sophisticated, is more acceptable.

The vast majority of our sample did not want any more children, and a majority claimed that they did not want their last child, but there was no evidence that the women who discontinued clinic attendance or method use were less likely to feel this way. Our conclusion to reject what we term 'simple rationality' throws further doubt upon the widespread view that such an association exists.

In common with many other parts of the world, the distribution system in Trinidad is dominated by health-related assumptions and controlled by the medical profession. There is reason to suppose that a sparse network of health clinics organised in the manner described may serve the interests of the staff and administrators more than the women themselves. Clinic factors did show some relationship with discontinuation and many women of all groups in our sample were inconvenienced by the clinics or doctors.

There is a strong case for 'demedicalising' family planning and we tend to support Nortman's conclusion that:

> ... professional adminstrators should administer the programmes so that they go beyond the limited maternal and child health approach, co-operate with the private sector to bring the services to the people and not the people to the services, train non-medical and paramedical personnel to dispense services, including the insertion of IUD's, introduce abortion on demand, (and) incorporate broad information and education campaigns ... (Nortman 1972, p. 18.)

More radically, some countries (e.g. Kenya and Sri Lanka) have adopted government-subsidised programmes to sell condoms commercially through small shopkeepers. These have led to increased use of condoms and greater acceptance of the ideas and legitimacy of family planning within the community. An additional important effect has been to integrate family planning into the everyday structure of society 'rather than (family planning) being injected into it through medical channels' (Black and Harvey, 1976, p. 107). Associated with this is the need to see contraceptive acceptors as people, not as 'clients' and least of all as 'patients'.

We conclude that rejection of the centrality of the medical profession within family planning programmes and of clinics as the point of distribution of supplies is not only necessary to spread family planning more widely, but that such an organisational structure and the pre-eminent position of doctors can be a negative influence on family planning programmes. The more services are re-organised in line with genuine consumer interests, the more they will approximate to the 'planning' goal of the programmes and, almost certainly, the more they will allow motivation to limit family size to be realised.

Notes

1. We would like to acknowledge a research grant from the IPPF (Western Hemisphere Region) and the co-operation of the Trinidad and Tobago Family Planning Association and National Family Planning Programme of the Trinidad and Tobago Government. We would also like to thank Dion McTair in Trinidad, Karin Janzon in London and Marie Elmer in Surrey, for their invaluable assistance.
2. The difference between our estimates and those of the Trinidad and Tobago Government and the FPA are partly due to the difficulty of collecting accurate data from numerous family planning clinics. This complexity is confounded by the fluid client careers which clients may have, e.g. a client can join the programme, so becoming a new acceptor, then stop attending and be defined as a 'drop-out'. The following year the client may re-attend the clinic for a few months and be defined as a 're-starter' only subsequently to terminate attendance and be defined as a 'drop-out' again. In addition, a proportion of new clients go to a clinic for advice and do not receive any family planning supplies. Rates of discontinuation will be inflated since the attenders may not have actually become family planning users yet are counted as such. For example, in the FPA 7.2 per cent of new attenders only received advice from the clinic they attended (FPA, 1975, p. 19).
3. For details of the methodology of this study see S. Arber, 'Sampling Procedure and Methodology', Appendix B of M. Cross (1976).
4. A woman using the IUD is defined as a 'drop-out' only when she has not returned for fifteen months after her last recorded visit. In addition, the reasons for discontinuation are likely to be different from those of clients on other methods, and the small numbers involved (under ten per cent of all clinic acceptors are IUD acceptors) would have been insufficient for separate analysis.
5. The average length of attendance for 'drop-outs' was approximately 40 per cent shorter than for a random sample of 'continuers'. It was expected that this differential length of use of clinics would affect the attitudes and clinic experience reported by the two groups. To prevent this, date of clinic registration was controlled in the design of the sample. The method of sample selection means that it is inappropriate to treat the total sample as representative of all attenders at Family Planning clinics in Trinidad.

References

Andrews, N. (1975), 'Trinidad and Tobago', in A. Segal (ed.), *Population Policies in the Caribbean* (Lexington, Mass, Lexington Books), pp. 73-87.
Berelson, B. (1966), 'KAP Studies on Fertility', in B. Berelson (ed.), *Family Planning and Population Programmes: A Review of World Developments* (Chicago, Univ. of Chicago Press).
Black, T. R. L. and Harvey, P. D. (1976), 'A Report on a Contraceptive Social Marketing Experiment in Rural Kenya', *Studies in Family Planning* 7(4), pp 101-8.
Blake, J. (1965), 'Demographic Science and the Redirection of Population Policy', *Journal of Chronic Diseases* 18, pp. 1181-1200.
Bone, M. (1975), *Meaures of Contraceptive Effectiveness and Their Uses*, Studies in Medical and Population Subjects, No. 28 (OPCS).
Burch, T. K. (1975), 'Theories of fertility as guides to population policy', *Social Forces* 54 (1), pp. 126-38.
Cisler, L. (1970), 'Unfinished business: birth control and women's liberation', in Morgan (ed.), *Sisterhood is Powerful* (N.Y., Vintage Books).
Cleland, J. (1973), 'A Critique of KAP Studies and some suggestions for their improvement', *Studies in Family Planning* 4 (2), pp. 42-47.
Commonwealth Caribbean (1974), *Population Census 1970* (Mona, Jamaica).
Coser, L. (1975), 'Two Methods in Search of a Substance', *American Sociological Review* 40 (6), pp. 691-700.
Cross, M. (1976), *Family Planning in Trinidad and Tobago: The Problem of Discontinuation* (University of Surrey, mimeo).
Davis, K. (1970a), 'Population Policy: Will Current Programme Succeed' in A. Bose *et al.* (Comp.), *Studies in Demography* (Chapel Hill, University of North Carolina Press).
   (1970b), *World Urbanization 1950-70 Volume I. Basic Data*, Population Monograph Series No. 4 (Berkeley, University of California).
Diggery, P. and McEwan, J. (1976), *Planning or Prevention? The New Face of 'Family Planning'* (London, Marion Boyars).
Family Planning Association (1975), *Medical Report, 1974* (Trinidad and Tobago).
Freedman, R. and Berelson, B. (1976), 'The Record of Family Planning Programs', *Studies in Family Planning* 7 (1), pp. 1-40.
Godwin, K. (1972), 'The Structure of Mass Attitudes in the United States and Latin America: Implications for Policy', in R. L. Clinton and R. K. Godwin (eds.), *Research in the Politics of Population* (Lexington, Mass., D.C. Heath and Co.) pp. 113-34.
   (1973), 'Methodology and Policy', in R. L. Clinton (ed.), *Population and Politics* (Lexington, Mass., Lexington Books), pp. 131-43.
Harewood, J. (1968), 'Recent Population Trends and Family Planning Activities in the Caribbean', *Demography* 5 (2), pp 874-93.
Harewood, J. and Abdulah, N. (1971), *Family Planning in Trinidad and Tobago in 1970* (Trinidad and Tobago, I.S.E.R.).
Hauser, P. (1970), 'On Non-Family Planning Methods of Population Control', in A. Bose *et al.* (Comp.), *Studies in Demography* (Chapel Hill, University of North Carolina Press), pp. 353-69.
Illich, I. (1973), *Celebration of Awareness: A Call for Institutional Revolution* (Harmondsworth, Penguin).
Kaiser, B. and Kaiser, I. (1974), 'The Challenge of the Women's Movement to American Gynaecology', *American Journal of Obstetrics and Gynaecology* 120 (5), pp. 652-61.
Kerr, C. B. (1972), 'Regional use and training of para-medical personnel', *Clinical Proceedings of the IPPF* (South East Asia and Oceania Regional

Medical and Scientific Congress, Sydney), pp. 29-37.
La Pierre, R. (1934), 'Attitudes Versus Actions', *Social Forces* 13, pp. 230-7.
McDonald, J. C. (1973), 'Unmet needs in Family Planning', unpublished paper presented to the IPPF International Conference, Brighton.
Mandle, J. (1973), *The Recent Decline in Fertility in Trinidad and Tobago* (University of California, Preliminary Paper No. 5, International Population and Urban Research).
Muller, C. (1974), 'Feminism, Society and Fertility Control', *Family Planning Perspectives* 6 (2), pp. 68-72.
Nortman, D. L. (1972),'Status of National Family Planning Programmes of Developing Countries in Relation to Demographic Targets', *Population Studies* 26, pp. 5-18.
Peel, J. and Potts, D.M. (1973), 'The Sociology of Population Control', *Social Science and Medicine* 7, pp. 179-90.
Potts, D. M. (1971), 'Family Planning in the Market Place', *Proceedings of the IPPF South East Asia and Oceania Regional Conference*, pp. 301-5.
Rich, W. (1973), *Smaller Families through Social and Economic Progress* (Washington, Overseas Development Council).
Scanzoni, J. and McMurray, M. (1972), 'Continuities in the Explanation of Fertility Control', *Journal of Marriage and the Family* 34 (2), pp. 315-21.
Segal, A. (ed.) (1975), *Population Policies in the Caribbean* (Lexington, Mass., Lexington Books).
Stimson, G. V. (1974), 'Obeying Doctors' Orders', *Social Science and Medicine* 8 (2), pp. 97-104.
Tietze, C. (1970), 'Ranking of Contraceptive Methods by levels of Effectiveness', *Advances in Planned Parenthood* Vol. VI (Amsterdam, Excerpta Medica), pp. 117-26.
Trinidad and Tobago (1974a), *Report on the Population Programme, 1973* (Ministry of Health).
  (1974b), *Population Abstract, 1960-1970* (Central Statistical Office).
  (1974c), *Population Census Bulletin No. 3 – Fertility* (Central Statistical Office).
  (1975), *Population and Vital Statistics, 1973 Report* (Central Statistical Office).
van Renselaar, J. R. (1974), 'The Adoption of Modern Birth Prevention Techniques in the Light of Social Control', in D. G. Jongmans and H. J. M. Claessen (eds.), *The Neglected Factor: Family Planning – Perceptions and Reactions at the Base* (Assen, Van Gorcum), pp. 67-89.
Viestra, G. A. (1974), 'Some Thoughts About the Attitude Concept in Relation to Family Planning', in D. G. Jongmans and H. J. M. Claessen (eds.), *The Neglected Factor: Family Planning – Perceptions and reactions at the base* (Assen, Van Gorcum), pp. 9-32.